50 Simple Thi
Do to Raise a C
Physica

Funds to purchase
this book were
provided by a
40th Anniversary Grant
from the
Foellinger Foundation.

ARCO

50 Simple Things You Can Do to Raise a Child Who Is Physically Fit

Joanne Landy, B.Ed. and
Keith Burridge, M.Ed., B.Ed.

Macmillan • USA

This book is dedicated to all the children of the world who exemplify the value of "play" in their daily lives. We need to learn from them!

Macmillan • USA
A Simon & Schuster Macmillan Company
1633 Broadway
New York, NY 10019-6785

Manufactured in the United States of America
10 9 8 7 6 5 4 3 2 1
Library of Congress Number: 97-071527
ISBN: 0-02-861984-6

Book design by Rachael McBrearty—Madhouse Productions

An Arco Book

Contents

Introduction

    To the Parents xi

    What Parents Need to Know xiii

    10 Essential Understandings xiii

Section 1   Understanding Fitness and Its Importance

The Health-Related Components Of Fitness 3

The Skill-Related Components of Fitness: 9

25 General Guidelines To Follow 10

Section 2   Coordination Activities—Body Management:
                  50 Fit Sessions

    Fit Session #1 17

    Fit Session #2 18

    Fit Session #3 20

    Fit Session #4 21

    Fit Session #5 23

    Fit Session #6 24

    Fit Session #7 27

    Fit Session #8 31

    Fit Session #9 34

    Fit Session #10 36

    Fit Session #11 38

Fit Session #12 41
Fit Session #13 44
Fit Session #14 47
Fit Session #15 50
Fit Session #16 52
Fit Session #17 55
Fit Session #18 57
Fit Session #19 60
Fit Session #20 63
Fit Session #21 65
Fit Session #22 67
Fit Session #23 70
Fit Session #24 73
Fit Session #25 76
Fit Session #26 79
Fit Session #27 81
Fit Session #28 83
Fit Session #29 85
Fit Session #30 87
Fit Session #31 89
Fit Session #32 92
Fit Session #33 95
Fit Session #34 98
Fit Session #35 101
Fit Session #36 104
Fit Session #37 106
Fit Session #38 109
Fit Session #39 112
Fit Session #40 114
Fit Session #41 117
Fit Session #42 120
Fit Session #43 122

Fit Session #44 124
Fit Session #45 126
Fit Session #46 127
Fit Session #47 128
Fit Session #48 130
Fit Session #49 132
Fit Session #50 133

Introduction

To the Parents

The content of this book is to provide you, the parents, with a variety of quality movement experiences that you and your child(ren) can do together. Acquiring competence and confidence in movement will enhance your child's overall coordination and nurture your child's self-esteem. Equally as important, your child will build up his/her fitness to develop good aerobic capacity, strength, flexibility, speed, agility, alertness, and reaction.

Children from an early age need to acquire good spatial awareness, both in personal and general space, develop body awareness (body image), and learn to move with effort and in relationship with others.

"Children need to learn to move, but at the same time, they need to move to learn."

Fundamental movement skills are the building blocks of all movement. They are the foundation for skills your child will use later in life to pursue recreational or competitive sporting activities. They include the locomotive movements of walking, running, dodging, jumping and landing, leaping, hopping, skipping, sliding, balancing, climbing, hanging, swinging, pushing, pulling, and rotating. Fundamental motor skills of rolling, throwing and catching, kicking, and striking can then be developed.

The established fact is that a child who is physically active from an early age and receives positive, enjoyable and successful movement experiences, will continue to engage in and pursue activity on a regular basis throughout his or her lifetime. The benefits in terms of "wellness" or general sense of well being are physiological, psychological (emotional stability), and academic. This book targets the 3–8 year old child and focuses on 50 of the best movement experiences you can do with your child. You will enjoy being actively involved too, and can benefit with quality time well invested in your child's welfare. These activities have been progressively organized with indoor and outdoor suggestions, including limited space or "rainy day" activities.

What Parents Need to Know

10 Essential Understandings

1. **Make fitness fun!**   How you as an adult look at fitness is different than how your child perceives "fitness." Children are not mini-adults. Children simply obtain their fitness by doing activities they enjoy. As soon as we as parents impose "training" on them, we are creating an uphill "battle of resistance." Young children's interests can be short term and quick changing. They have an inconsistent attention span. They tire easily, but recover quickly. Be reasonable in the degree of physical exertion required.

2. **Everyone plays!**   "Play" is fundamental to life and contributes to the overall development of your child. Play is a significant means for your child to explore, express, and discover many aspects of life. "Play" can also help your child learn and find real value and meaning in the experience, develop fitness and skills, and learn "social graces."

3. **Understand the "Want-Fear" premise.**   We as adults work on our fitness out of "fear" of a heart attack, of gaining weight, and acquiring hypokinetic diseases of a modern civilization. Some of us engage in fitness workouts because we do indeed enjoy activity as a lifestyle pursuit;

others become addicted, even obsessive. But children are too detached from the "fear" factor; therefore, we as parents need to develop the "want to" attitude at an early age, and this is achieved by always making activity an enjoyable event for them.

4. **Know the importance of Body Management.** From an early age children need to develop an appreciation and awareness of their bodies and what they can do in a "child-like" way. Children who are poorly coordinated or lack general overall coordination will not develop good fitness. These children do not have appropriate movement skills. For example, a child who can't run or who doesn't run properly, who keeps falling over or running into things and getting hurt, is hindered significantly in his/her aerobic development.

   Children need to be able to manage their bodies. A prerequisite to any fitness or activity program is that children feel comfortable with moving. A child who doesn't like to be active because movement is difficult for him/her will have a tendency to become overweight and lethargic, and have poor aerobic endurance and coordination problems. Overweight children, children who lack coordination, and children who lack flexibility will look for excuses to be inactive. This has significant implications for his/her growth and development, general fitness, and social development. Therefore, we must impact early—with fun, enjoyable "coordination" activities.

5. **Be aware of kids' growth and development.** Your child's bones have not developed to maturity. Movement is needed for development of strong bones and muscles; therefore, it is important that your child experience developmentally appropriate activities for his/her age group.

6. **Be a positive role model.** Children learn by example. Your children learn by watching you. They will mimic your actions, whether you are a cycling enthusiast or a "couch potato" TV addict. Be a positive role model by being enthusiastic and "joining in" whenever and wherever possible.

Your child needs your approval. Encourage, praise, and provide constructive feedback, but don't push or become overbearing.

7. **See FITNESS as the "big" picture.**   Fitness needs to be viewed as a holistic experience. The important point to emphasize is that physical fitness is only one part of health and well-being, which also includes: nutrition, "play," mental health, quality sleep, relaxation, and emotional health. For a child to be functioning at his/her optimal pace, there must be a balance of all these components. They are all "life keys" in the big picture.

Physical fitness is developed from exercise and activity, but physical fitness needs to be partnered with good nutrition. Both exercise and good nutrition contribute to overall health—one without the other creates an imbalance. Thus:

General Physical Health = Regular Exercise + Good Nutrition

Physical Fitness has 2 components:

Health-Related	*Skill-Related*
Cardiovascular	Agility
Flexibility	Balance
Muscular Strength	Coordination
Muscular Endurance	Power
Body Composition	Speed
	Reaction Time

Health-Related components focus on developing good health and preventing diseases and other problems resulting from inactivity (hypokinetic diseases). **Skill-related components** focus on learning skills and developing the ability to perform well in overall movement, sports, dance, and gymnastics.

8. **Be aware of exercise "do's" and "don'ts."**   Always "warm up" your child first with low to moderate activity. Movements should be gentle and rhythmical, then gradually increased in intensity. Try to use all the major muscle groups in the warm-up activity.

    Never stretch "cold" muscles. Avoid ballistic movements when stretching. Avoid exercises that hyperextend any joint areas. No massive weight-bearing exercises should be used. Children can use their own body weight to develop strength.

9. **Provide a variety of activities.**   Make activity the "name of the game," but vary the intensity. Make the activity fun, interesting, stimulating, and motivating!

10. **Develop a "knowing" attitude and an exercise habit.**   You need to develop a knowing attitude, not necessarily a "fitness" attitude. Get your child used to being active, used to doing exercise, and "in the know" of *why* exercise is so good for you.

Consistency becomes a habit. You need to establish with your child an activity routine schedule. But don't mistake consistency with regularity. You may not always have the time or the opportunity to do an activity session with your child at the same time each day, so be realistic about the time constraints and be flexible within consistency.

SECTION 1

Understanding Fitness and Its
Importance

We need to reinforce the values of exercise in an age-appropriate way to our children. It is not just the "doing" of the exercise or activity, but the developing of a "knowing" attitude that is so important. Children need to realize that you cannot "store" fitness like you can store food in a fridge or money in a bank. Fitness/activity must be a regular occurrence—ideally daily! You need to observe your children at play and take a "mental snapshot" of their activity level. Are they generally active throughout the activity session? Do they show through body language (facial expressions) enjoyment of what they are doing? Do they express verbally their excitement and "fun" in what they are doing?

The **F.I.T.T. Principle** (F— Frequency; I—Intensity; T—Time; and T—Type) states that we need to spend at least 3 times per week in on-going, continuous activity of at least 20-30 minutes in duration, in our target heart range. A variety of activities such as walking, jogging, swimming and water exercises, cycling, dancing, roller-blading, different sporting activities (basketball, tennis, soccer), rope jumping, cross-country skiing, hiking, gardening, or canoeing, is recommended instead of just engaging in one type of activity. Variety also allows different muscle groups to be used and other muscle groups not to be over-used.

The Health-Related Components Of Fitness

Cardiovascular (CV) Fitness

1. Cardiovascular (CV) Fitness has to do with the efficient working of the heart-lung systems to supply fuel—oxygen—to the working muscles. CV fitness requires a strong heart muscle. The heart muscle becomes stronger through exercise just like other muscles of the body. Therefore, it is important that the heart be exercised regularly from an early age; otherwise, it will never work as efficiently as it should. A strong healthy heart that increases in size and power can pump more blood with each beat and therefore, for any given amount of work (as well as at rest), the heart rate will be lower. This tells us that our heart is not working as strenuously as an unfit heart.

Heart rate (pulse) is important to determine if a person is doing enough exercise (intensity). The average resting heart rate of a child is about 80 beats per minute; an adult between 70–80 beats per minute; but a trained athlete's heart rate can be in the low 50s!

Aerobic exercise is activity for which the body can supply adequate oxygen to the working muscles to sustain activity for a long time. This produces cardiovascular fitness. Regular exercise reduces the risk of heart disease by building CV fitness; burning off calories helps to control body fatness and to develop muscular endurance.

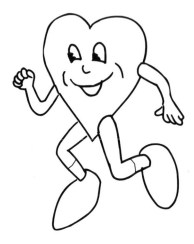

Practice Activity 1: "The Heart Workout"

Have the child move in different ways to your signals: walk; power walk; walk with quick changes of direction; walk on toes; walk on heels; walk backwards; march; march changing direction every 4 steps; jog straight ahead; jog with quick changes of direction; skip happily along; slide-step keeping low and moving in different directions. On the signal "Freeze!" have the child put one hand against his/her chest (left hand side) and listen to his/her heart. Let the other hand open and close to show this pulse beat.

Practice Activity 2: "Pulse Beat"

Listen to your heart beating by placing your 2nd and 3rd fingers on either side of the Adam's apple (carotid artery) and count the number of beats in 30 seconds. Multiply by 2 to get the beats per minute (b.p.m.) *or* place your 2nd and 3rd fingers just below the base of the thumb on the wrist to locate the radial artery.

Flexibility

2. Flexibility is the range of motion around a joint. This component of fitness is the most neglected of the 5 health-related components. Developing good flexibility can help prevent injury, muscle strain, muscle spasms and soreness, shin splints, and backache, as well as keep muscles toned, improve spinal mobility, and maintain joint suppleness.

As children grow older their flexibility increases until they become adolescents when they become progressively less flexible. Generally, girls tend to be more flexible than boys. Some children have a high degree of flexibility. We say that they are "double-jointed," but correctly their unusual flexibility is a genetic trait that makes their joints "hypermobile."

Research suggests that muscles need to be stretched to about 10% beyond their normal length to bring about improved flexibility. The result of a joint not being moved regularly through its full range of motion is a shortening of muscles and ligaments. Lack of use, injury (body part immobilized by a cast), poor posture, and poor working postures, can result in loss of flexibility in a fairly short time. Thus flexibility needs to be a daily occurrence!

Before performing an aerobic activity, static stretching (stretching slowly and holding for a certain time, 10+ seconds) should be used in the warm-up and cool-down." Remember the general rule: stretch the area that you strengthen, as well as strengthening the area that you stretch."

Remember these precautions as well:

- ⚽ Avoid ballistic-type stretching—use slow gentle stretching, through the whole range of motion, or hold static stretches for at least 10 seconds.
- ⚽ Don't stretch a muscle until it becomes painful—pain is no gain!
- ⚽ Don't overstretch weak muscles.
- ⚽ Don't stretch any swollen joints.

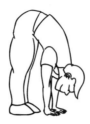

Practice Activity: "Good Morning, Wakie, Wakie" Stretch

- ⚽ In your own space stretch your arms up to the sky.
- ⚽ Raise up on your toes as you stretch upwards.
- ⚽ Let your eyes follow your hands.
- ⚽ Circle your arms in towards the middle making large circles.
- ⚽ Now circle your arms away from the middle.
- ⚽ Gently turn from side to side, pushing the hand out to the opposite side.
- ⚽ Shake all over like a wet dog coming out of the water.
- ⚽ Slowly sink to the floor into back-lying position.
- ⚽ Raise one leg, holding it at the ankle with both hands; keep it straight and gently press it towards your head. Repeat with the other leg.
- ⚽ In back-lying position, do a "Pencil" stretch, extending arms overhead and hold for 10 seconds.
- ⚽ Do "Angels in the Snow," then another Pencil Stretch.

Muscular Strength

3. Muscular Strength is measured by the amount of force you can exert with a single maximum effort. Good muscular strength helps to increase work effort, to decrease the chance of injury, to prevent back injury and poor posture, to improve athletic performance, and perhaps even to save a life. Through improving your child's muscular strength, the strength of bones, tendons, and ligaments are also increased. Children whose bones are still growing need to have low-impact exercises; otherwise, the result could be permanent growth-stunting damage to the growth plates.

You need to discuss with your child the importance of having strong arm muscles: to carry out daily work and play, such as taking out the garbage, bringing in the groceries, raking the lawn, throwing a football, hanging and swinging on playground apparatus, swimming in the surf, and meeting unforeseen emergencies.

Power is a combination of strength and speed and is both health-related and skill-related.

Practice Activity: "Animal Walks"

Have child perform different "animal walks" such as:

Crab Walk Greeting: Greet your child on all fours, face upwards, by lifting one foot upwards and "shaking" the foot of your child's. Repeat "shaking" with the other foot.

Puppy Dog Walk: On all fours, hands and feet, walk like a puppy dog. Now walk like a lame puppy dog who has an injured back foot.

Kicking Bronco: From the squat position, take weight on your hands and kick your feet upwards into the air.

Seal Walk: In front-lying position, take weight only on your hands and drag your feet behind you as you move along.

Clock Walk: In front support position, keep your feet in the center of the "clock" and walk your hands to 3 o'clock, 9 o'clock, 12 o'clock, and so on.

Inchworm: From front support position, walk your feet up to your hands, then walk your hands away from your feet. Keep repeating this pattern as you "inch" along the floor.

Muscular Endurance

4. Muscular Endurance has to do with the muscle's ability to continue to contract over a long period. Good muscular endurance gives you the ability to repeat a movement without getting tired or to hold a position or carry something for a long period of time without being fatigued. A child who has good muscular endurance will enjoy and have greater success in his/her daily work activities, in play, and in sporting and athletic competitions.

Practice Activity: Playground Fun

Hand-Walk: Have your child "hand-walk" across the high bar.

Bar Swing and Hangs: On the high bar, hang upside down; travel across with your hands and feet.

Curl-Ups: In hook-lying position, cross hands on shoulders. Curl up until shoulders are off the floor, the slowly roll down to starting position. Repeat.

Rope Jumping: On the spot.

Body Composition

5. Body Composition has to do with the relative percentage of fat, bone, muscle, and other tissues that make up the body.

Body fatness (either overfat or underfat) can lead to health concerns including degenerative diseases such as diabetes and heart disease, and can even shorten life span. Skin fold califers are used to precisely measure body fat; however, you can generally observe overfatness (or underfatness) in your child. The important factor is that you observe and monitor your child's diet, eating habits, and nutritional intake, as well as his/her activity level.

The Skill-Related Components of Fitness

Agility, balance, coordination, power, speed, and **reaction time** are considered to be the main components of skill-related physical fitness.

- **Agility** is the ability to quickly and accurately change direction of your body movement in general space. Examples: downhill skiing and wrestling.

- **Balance** is the ability to maintain body equilibrium while on the spot or while moving. Examples: moving on a balance beam and waterskiing.

- **Coordination** is the ability control body part movements in order to perform motor tasks well and accurately. Examples: juggling, baseball batting, hitting a golf ball, kicking a ball, and striking a ball with a racquet.

- **Power** is the ability to quickly transfer energy into force. Examples: throwing a shot put and throwing a javelin.

- **Speed** is the ability to perform a movement quickly. Example: running the 100m sprint.

- **Reaction Time** is the ability to respond quickly to a stimulation. Example: starting a sprint race or being a racing car driver.

25 General Guidelines to Follow

1. Make activity a family affair.

2. Set an example yourself—be a good role model.

3. Turn the television off. Just to encourage them to go outside is promoting fitness.

4. Develop regularity and habit in doing activity. Produce a timetable but make it flexible and adaptable.

5. Be aware of your child's physical capabilities.

6. Develop posture. Check and reinforce good posture.

7. Foster good sleeping habits.

8. Develop good eating habits.

9. Encourage drinking water each day. Water is essential. Talk about dehydration and its effects.

10. Develop spatial awareness—general and personal.

11. Develop body awareness and memory awareness.

12. Develop a good sense of balance.

13. Develop aerobic capacity.

14. Develop upper body strength.

15. Develop mid-body toning.

16. Develop lower body strength.

17. Develop reaction and alertness.

18. Develop flexibility—upper body.

19. Develop flexibility—lower body.

20. Develop agility—quickness.

21. Develop speed.

22. Develop good range of vision—peripheral vision.

23. Develop hand-eye coordination.

24. Develop foot-eye coordination.

25. Do relaxation activities.

10 Strategies to Encourage the Reluctant Child

1. Observe WHY your child is reluctant: Is he/she overweight, insecure? Does he/she have poor coordination, low self-esteem, a fear of failure? Does he/she feel unsafe?

2. Create a safe, fun, positive environment. Ensure that there is absolutely no physical threat, no ridicule, no bullying, no put-downs. No "emotional hurts."

3. Provide feedback that is instantaneous—at the "time of doing." Give praise and encouragement; words such as: "I loved the way you did that!"; "I'm so proud of you—you ran all the way!"

4. Try to experience success within a short period of time.

5. Offer some kind of incentive or reward sometimes. Instant reward is praise and encouragement. A reward could follow a goal: "after we go cycling together, we will go to the movies."

6. Keep within the limits of your child's abilities. Don't force him/her or constantly be at him/her. Ideally, we would like your child to take responsibility for his/her own activity.

7. Don't be overprotective.

8. Don't confuse a child's needs with his/her wants. A young child doesn't have the experience or knowledge to know what is good for them. For example, the child who consistently says to the parent, "I don't want to go outside to play, I would rather watch TV." is expressing a "want" not a "need." In this situation, as a caring adult we need to impose our knowledge of the importance of exercise on the child and encourage or even insist that he/she goes out to play regularly.

9. Establish firmness and consistency. Insist that you will do an activity together and stick to it.

10. Vary the activities that you do with your child to sustain his/her interest.

Coordination Activities— Body Management:

50 Fit Sessions

Now we're ready to get you "in motion." Before we start with the activities, just remember that children need to develop the skills and positive attitude to *want* to be active. As parents it is our responsibility to encourage and help develop the habit of regular exercise. This is far more important than trying to train a child to achieve a heart rate of 150 beats per minute over 30 minutes of exercise. (This is an adult's perspective of exercise, not a child's!)

We are introducing only 50 suggestions to get your child physically fit. There are literally thousands of ideas. Perhaps each of these 50 ways are just the "seeds" of more ideas you can generate. Enjoy and grow with your child!

Fit Session #1:
Spatial Awareness Activities

Children need to understand spatial language both physically and verbally so they can successfully and confidently move around in their personal space and general space. Say the following tasks and observe how they respond. (Be sure to make note of any difficulties your child may have.)

- Stand in front of the chair; sit behind the ball; kneel next to the ball.
- Move onto the bench, then jump off; stand up, sit down.
- Travel under a stick, now go over.
- Move along the rope; travel between the ladder rungs.
- Run around the tree; move through the big tire.
- Stand face to face; now back to back, then beside, behind.
- Be high, be low; roll along the ground.
- Move in a big circle; make your circle become smaller and smaller, larger and larger (repeat with triangles, squares).
- Skip forwards; walk backwards; slide sideways; jump from side to side, forwards and backwards; hop straight ahead.

Fit Session #2:
Body Awareness Activities

Children need to have an understanding of their own bodies. They need to know their body parts and where they are in relation to each other, including left and right "sidedness." Use the following body and directional language and observe how your child responds. Emphasize good posture whenever possible, observe, and offer comment.

- ⚽ Have your child point to the body part you name, first with eyes open, then with eyes closed. Repeat, having him/her point and name the body part.

- ⚽ Trace an outline of your child's body in back-lying position either on a large piece of paper or with chalk on tarmac. Then have him/her fill in the details.

- ⚽ Ask your child to: "snap your fingers"; "blink your eyes"; "turn your head from side to side"; "stamp your feet"; "point your elbows upwards"; "wiggle your bottom"; shake all over.

- ⚽ Stand tall. Sit tall. Back straight, head up, eyes looking forward. Walk "tall." Balance a beanbag on your head as you walk.

- ⚽ Now try directional actions such as: open and close your right hand; lift your left knee; raise your right elbow; circle your right arm; balance on your left foot; touch your right knee to your left elbow; hold your left foot with your right hand . . .

⚽ Have your child in standing position, cross arms and legs, right over left and sit down, then stand up again without undoing this body position. Repeat, crossing left over right arms and legs.

Fit Session #3:
Motor Memory Activities

Motor memory has to do with your child's ability to visually and auditorily copy single movements, movement patterns, and rhythm patterns. Begin with just one movement and then increase according to one movement for each year old. At first the child may just remember the moves in any order, but strive for correct sequencing of the moves. Playground equipment in your backyard or local park is ideal for "memory touch" activities.

- ⚽ Have child copy hand movements: palms up, palms down, hands up, hands down, hands sideways.

- ⚽ Have child copy body movements: arm circling, hands on head, knee lifts, seat circles, leg shakes, different facial expressions . . .

- ⚽ Have child copy clapping rhythms: finger-snapping, foot-stamping, hand-clapping, hand- and foot-clapping.

- ⚽ Have child "touch" different body parts in order: hand–knee–toe; touch 3 different objects: chair–table–door; elbow to fence, nose to tree, shoulder to swing.

- ⚽ Play "Follow-the-Leader" around the playground.

- ⚽ Play "Simon Says" in which child only does the movements if you first say "Simon says, jump up and down. Now turn around." (Child does not "turn around," but continues "jumping up and down.")

Fit Session #4:
Balancing Activities

Your child may need some support when doing these balancing activities. Try to get them to "feel" their body position by closing their eyes. Each balance should be held for 10 seconds and repeated at least 3 times until you observe that your child has control.

- Balance on 1 foot, with your hands out to the sides. Hold for 10 second count. Balance on the other foot. Hold for 10 second count. Repeat, but with eyes closed.

- How many different ways can you balance on your: front (upper/lower torso) of your body, backside of your body, either side of your body? Try with eyes closed.

- Balance on different body combinations: 1 hand and 1 foot; 1 knee, 1 foot, 1 elbow; 2 knees, head . . .

- Balance on a line; a bench; a balance board; a beam.

- Walk with arms out to sides along the beam. Kneel, stand up, turn around, small jumps, catch a ball and walk along the beam.

- Make a bridge using different body parts: 1 leg and 2 hands (3 body part balance).

- Make a partner balance. How many different balancing positions can you make?

⚽ Move around until you hear me call "Statue!" and a number. Then make a balance on (3) body parts and hold for 5 seconds.

⚽ Make up a balance of your own!

Fit Session #5:
Starting and Stopping Activities

Your child needs to learn how to control his/her body at an early age so that he/she will not get physically hurt and his/her confidence will continue to improve, as well as his/her alertness, reaction, and listening ability to respond quickly. These skills may even save your child's life in a threatening situation. Observe your child when he/she stops—is he/she in control? Does he/she fall over? Does he/she stop immediately? Offer good praise and encouragement.

- ⚽ Have your child run in general space, changing directions often. On your signal "Freeze!," the child stops immediately.

- ⚽ Repeat having your child move in different ways: walking, hopping, skipping, jogging, sliding, moving backwards, moving on all fours . . .

- ⚽ Have your child run for 5 seconds, then "jump-stop" (both feet touch the ground at the same time, feet are shoulder-width apart, knees bent).

- ⚽ Use music to start and stop your child.

- ⚽ With a partner, have one partner follow the other like a "shadow." On signal "Freeze!", both come to a jump-stop. If the partner behind can touch the partner in front, change roles. Continue in this way.

Fit Session #6

Walking is an ideal "warm-up" activity to get children moving. Young and old can participate together in a variety of walking environments.

Fit Activity #1   Fit Focus: Cardiovascular

Walking Activities

As your child's fitness increases, gradually speed up the pace of the activities. Remember to use "Freeze!" as your stopping signal.

- ⚽ Walk forwards, backwards, sideways.
- ⚽ Walk on toes, on heels.
- ⚽ Walk quickly, slowly, quick changes of direction, change of pace.
- ⚽ Take big steps, baby steps, feet close together, feet wide apart.
- ⚽ Walk in straight, curved, and zigzag lines, and in figure-eight, circular, and rectangular shapes.
- ⚽ Walk happily, sadly, angrily, excited, frightened.
- ⚽ Walk to music with a steady 4/4 beat.
- ⚽ Do marching steps and clap hands in time to music.

Games

⚽ **Follow-the-Leader:** use the above activities.

⚽ **Here, Where, There:** On "Here"—walk towards you; on "Where"—walk on the spot; on "There"—walk away from you.

⚽ **Memory Walk:** give child 3 or 4 walking tasks to do in the order given or do in any order. Ask child to listen carefully before moving. Examples:

> Walk to touch 3 lines, walk to touch 2 opposite walls, walk to touch 2 circles . . .

> Walk to touch 3 trees, then walk to touch around the playground equipment, walk under 2 objects . . .

> Take your dog for a walk to the park or beach.

Fit Activity #2   Fit Focus: Strength

Find a local park with a playground station with lots of interesting apparatus. Encourage your child to explore all parts of it: hanging, climbing, swinging, balancing, sliding. When your child is performing inverted hanging activities (hanging by the legs) let your child take her body weight, but always take the precaution of hanging on to the child.

Challenge your child by saying things like:

⚽ Can you hang for 10 seconds while I count 1, 2, 3? . . .

⚽ Show me how you can climb to the top. Careful!

⚽ Can you swing across on the "flying fox"?

⚽ How many different ways can you move down the slide?

Fit Activity #3   Fit Focus: Flexibility

Dead Ant Stretch

- Pretend you're a "dead ant" and lie on your back with your feet and hands in the air. Holding your ankles and keeping your legs straight, gently stretch towards your head.
- Stretch by holding opposite hand to opposite ankle.
- Repeat using other hand. (Can use right and left terms.)

Angels in the Snow

- In back-lying position, spread your legs and arms apart, then together. Now just open your legs apart; then just arms.
- Repeat with just one side moving away; then other side.

Fit Tip

You have about 600 muscles in your body. Your heart is the most important muscle in your body. It is about the size of your fist and located underneath your breast bone.

Fit Session #7

Children, in general, like to move quickly. Remind them to watch where they are going to avoid collisions.

Fit Activity #1   Fit Focus: Cardiovascular

(Remember to use the stopping signal "Freeze!")

Running Activities

- Jog on the spot; jog straight ahead.
- Jog along the outside boundary of the basketball court.
- Jog slowly; jog quickly; jog changing speed on your signal.
- Run with quick changes of direction (dodging) on your signal.
- Jog up the hill; jog down the hill.
- Jog in a large rectangular path, power-walking the short sides and running as fast as you can along the long sides.
- Jog in a big figure-eight.
- Jog in time to the music, changing direction every 8 beats, and clapping your hands when you change direction.
- Jog lightly; jog heavily.
- Run as fast as you can for 10 seconds; then walk 10 seconds. Repeat this pattern.
- Jog to touch the objects that I name: tree, fence, goal post, line.

Games

⚽ **Activity Lines:** Mark off 4 lines that are spaced 10 yards/meters apart. Jog forward to the first line; jog backwards to the starting line; jog forwards to the second line; jog backwards to the starting line; jog forwards to the third line, and then again backwards to start. How fast can you do this?

⚽ **Follow Me Jog:** This can be done in a playground area. Just have your child follow you around the playground, around trees, over and under obstacles, off and on obstacles.

Fit Activity #2   Fit Focus: Strength

Combative Play

Combative play is a "friendly contact" play in which children either push or pull against each other.

⚽ Stand facing your child, with one foot slightly forward and knees bent. Let your child push against the palms of your hands.

⚽ **Tug-o-War:** Using a finger grip and pulling against each other. Use right hands, then left hands.

⚽ **Towel Tug-o-War:** Use a towel gripped in both hands, pull against each other.

⚽ **Hoppo Bumpo:** Stand on one leg facing each other with arms crossed. Each partner tries to "bump" the other partner off-balance.

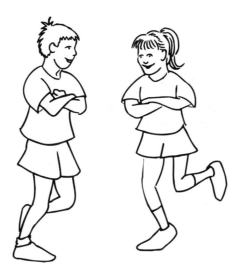

Fit Activity #3   Fit Focus: Flexibility

Head & Eye Stretch

Let your eyes look in one direction as your head turns gently from one side to the other. Keep your head still as your eyes look upwards, then downwards, to one side, to the other side. Let your eyes trace a large circle in front of you; a figure-eight.

Belly-Button Swivels

Standing tall, with your feet shoulder-width apart, trace a large circle with your belly button. Keeping your upper body still, circle your lower body 4 times one way, then circle 4 times the other way.

Fit Tip

Your resting heart rate as a child is about 80 beats per minute. Listen to your heart beat after you have been moving around quickly. Feel the pulse at your chest or near your Adam's apple. Open and close your fist to show how fast your heart is beating.

Fit Session #8

This session is a progression from walking to jogging to running in different patterns, yet under control.

Fit Activity #1   Fit Focus: Cardiovascular

Running Activities

- ⚽ **Zigzag Running:** Set out about 6 markers 2–3 yards/meters apart. Have your child zigzag between the markers and return. Ask them to travel in different ways: forwards, sideways by slide-stepping, and backwards; power walking . . .

- ⚽ **Triangle Running:** Set the markers in a triangular pattern, spaced 6 meters apart, and marked #1, #2, and #3. Have your child start at #1 marker, run around #2 marker, back around #1, then around #3 marker, back around #1. Repeat this circuit twice.

- ⚽ **Rectangle Running:** Mark out a rectangle that is 6 meters by 10 meters. Have your child run the lengths of the rectangle, and walk the widths. Repeat running in the opposite direction.

- ⚽ **Changing Speed:** Space 4 markers at 10 meters apart. Have your child run quickly to the first marker; slowly to the next; quickly to the next; and slowly to the finish. Repeat.

⊛ **Partner Tail Tag:** Play a game of "chasey" with your child by trying to pull his tail (flag or long piece of cloth tucked into the back of his/her shorts). Take turns being "IT."

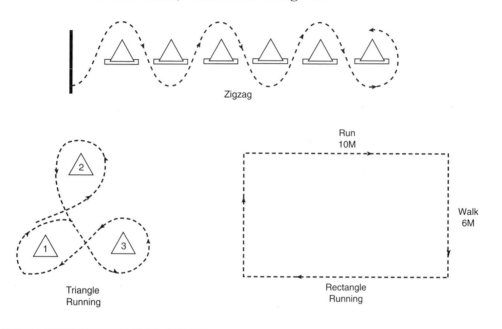

Zigzag

Triangle
Running

Rectangle
Running

Fit Activity #2   Fit Focus: Strength

Parachute Play

Use a beach towel, a 6-foot parachute, or a used sheet.

⊛ Place a small object such as a soft ball, bean bag, a small soft toy and shake the object up and down on the towel.

⊛ **Popcorn:** Shake several light objects off the towel.

- ⚽ Plant your feet and at the same time, pull away from the towel. Repeat with your back to the towel.

- ⚽ Slide-step in a circle holding onto the towel and leaning away.

- ⚽ Make up another activity to do with your towel. Example: Roll up towel, plant your feet, and have a "tug-o-war."

Fit Activity #3   Fit Focus: Flexibility

Stretching Shapes

Name a shape then have your child hold that shape for 5 –10 seconds. Examples:

- ⚽ A wide shape—like the letter "Y" or "T"

- ⚽ A round shape—like a ball

- ⚽ A long shape—like a pencil

- ⚽ A curved shape—like the letter "S" or a banana

- ⚽ A twisted shape—like a pretzel

- ⚽ your turn . . .

Fit Tip

Your *biceps* are the muscles of your upper arm. They are needed to help you lift and carry things, to throw objects, to swim, to use the parachute!

Fit Session #9

Fit Activity #1   Fit Focus: Cardiovascular

Children love games in which they can "make believe" and use their imagination.

- Move like a prancing horse.
- Move like a speed boat or jet ski, cutting through the waves.
- Move like an ice skater or a figure skater.
- Move like a magpie swooping down on a small critter.
- Move like a Boeing 747 taking off down the runway.
- Move like a kite dipping and lifting in the air.
- Move like a lawn mower cutting the grass.
- Move like a busy bee flitting from flower to flower.

Fit Activity #2   Fit Focus: Strength

Shadow Boxer

Pretend you're a boxer. Show me how you can punch into the air. Make your feet "dance."

Karate Kid

Use your arms to slash through the air; your feet to kick.

Bucking Bronco

Take your weight on your hands and kick your feet into the air.

Fit Activity #3   Fit Focus: Flexibility

Sunflower

Begin curled up into a tight ball. Slowly start to uncurl and open up to a standing position with your arms in the air. Take a 10 second count to end on tip toes. Now take 10 seconds to return to a tight curled position as low to the ground as you can go. Repeat.

Fit Tip

Your *triceps* are your muscles underneath your upper arm. They are your basketball-shooting muscles, and help you do a forward roll.

Fit Session #10

Fit Activity #1   Fit Focus: Cardiovascular

Shallow Water Activities (about knee- or waist-deep)

- ⚽ Face your child on opposite sides of the pool. Walk across the pool to change places.
- ⚽ Repeat but this time zigzag your way across the pool.
- ⚽ Hold a kick board and walk across the pool.
- ⚽ Repeat the above activities, jogging across the pool.
- ⚽ Throw a ball forward, walk (jog) to it. Repeat.
- ⚽ Hold your child while he/she flutter kicks legs in the water, making as much "splash" as possible.
- ⚽ Have your child hold onto the edge of the pool and make as much splash as possible.
- ⚽ Holding your child's hands, jump up and down in the water, in a circle, change directions; jump forwards; jump backwards; from side to side.
- ⚽ Repeat, but hop on 1 foot in the water, then the other, changing hopping foot every 4 hops.

Fit Activity #2   Fit Focus: Strength

- ⚽ Holding your child in the water have him do the front crawl stroke; breaststroke; backstroke; treading water.
- ⚽ Push a beachball down into the water and make it "bob" up!
- ⚽ Hand paddle on a small floating board.

Fit Activity #3   Fit Focus: Flexibility

- ⚽ Holding your child, face upwards, in the water, let him make a wide floating shape ("star").
- ⚽ Hanging onto the edge, have your child lean away, stretching out as much as possible; gently open and close legs.
- ⚽ Standing in water, gently push the water, "slow-motion" treading.
- ⚽ Make up your own "water stretch!"

Fit Tip

When you move in water, you are buoyant, which puts little stress on the joints of your body.

Fit Session #11

Children love to play "chasey" or tag-type games. Remind them to watch where they are going so they avoid collisions.

Fit Activity #1   Fit Focus: Cardiovascular

Running & Dodging Activities

- ⚽ **Shadow Dodging Game:** Stand in front of your child. On your "GO!" signal, have your child follow you like a "shadow" around the play area as you make quick changes of direction (dodging). On STOP, both of you come to an immediate stop. If your child can touch you by taking a giant pivot step towards you, (one foot must stay in contact with the floor), then change roles.

  Use a variety of locomotion movements: walking, running, skipping, hopping, slide-stepping, etc. Praise good "stops!"

- ⚽ **Chasey:** Decide who is "IT!" and how IT will tag you. (Suggest pulling a flag from the back of your shorts, or touching you with a soft ball, or throwing a beanbag to hit you below your knees.) When IT makes the tag, you become IT and give chase.

- ⚽ **What Time Is It, Mr. Wolf?:** Have your child stand at the end of a play area you've marked out. Each time your child asks "What time is it, Mr. Wolf?," you answer by giving a specific time such as

"3 o'clock." Your child must then take 3 giant steps towards you. When you answer "Dinnertime," give chase trying to tag your child before he safely crosses over the endline.

Fit Activity #2   Fit Focus: Strength

- **Bridges & Tunnels:** Make a bridge by taking your weight on your hands and feet, while your child moves through the tunnel. Then reverse roles. Explore different ways of doing this.

- **Leap Frog:** Take up a low position on all fours, tucking your head down. Have child "leap frog" over your back to land in the same position as you. Then you leap frog over your child. Continue along in this way. How many leap-frogs can you do?

- **Ski Jumps:** Holding hands with your child and standing on the same side of a line, jump together from side-to-side.

Fit Activity #3   Fit Focus: Flexibility

- **Tick-Tock:** Stand back-to-back with your child and interlock fingers. Gently lean to one side, bending knees, and touch pointer finger to the ground ("tick"). Straighten, then lean to other side to do the same ("tock").

- **Churn-the-Butter:** Face your child and, holding hands, turn in one direction, under raised arms away from each other, back-to-back, and continue turning to face again. Repeat in the other direction.

You have 206 bones in your body. Your bones support and protect the parts inside. Remember to watch where you are going when traveling with quick changes of direction!

Fit Session #12

Ropes are inexpensive pieces of equipment that can be used in an area with limited space.

Fit Activity #1   Fit Focus: Cardiovascular

Rope Jumping Activities

For short rope activities, select a rope length for yourself and for your child so that when you step into the center of the rope, the handles come just under arms, but no higher than the top of the shoulders.

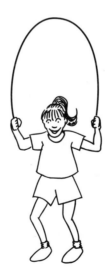

⚽ **Rope Patterns:** Lay a rope straight along the ground and have your child jump in a zigzag pathway from one end to the other. Jump from side to side. Then be a "tightrope walker" along rope.

Make a circle with your rope and your child's. Play a game of "Circle Tag" around the rope. Leap over the circle rope in different ways. Run and take off on 1 foot, to land with 2 feet in the circle.

⚽ **Long Rope Jumping:** Using a long rope, with one end tied to a fence or post, have child stand in the center and swing rope gently under his/her feet. Cue child when to jump, "Jump-Jump-Jump!"

As rope jumping ability improves, challenge child to keep jumping as long as possible. Jump and turn around; jump opening and closing feet; jump and clap hands or snap fingers; jump and bounce a ball. What other challenges can you do? Run in "front door" to jump in center of rope, and run out.)

Gradually, increase speed and duration.

⚽ **Short Rope Jumping:** (Once your child has developed good rhythm jumping in a long rope, then use a short rope.)

Make up "Jumping Jingles."

Hot Pepper—How many jumps can be made in 30 seconds; 45 seconds; 1 minute?

Fit Activity #2   Fit Focus: Strength

Rope Circling

Hold handles of rope together in one hand. Try the following activities with one hand, then the other.

- ☢ **Helicopters:** Circle rope overhead. Can you make it "sing"?
- ☢ **Propellers:** Circle rope in front of you. Make it sing.
- ☢ **Wheelies:** Circle rope with your right hand on right side; switch to your left hand and circle rope on left side.
- ☢ **Twisters:** Circle rope in front in a figure-eight pattern.
- ☢ **Strong Hands:** Fold rope in half and then again in half. Holding firmly onto ends try to pull rope apart for a 10 second count.

Fit Activity #3   Fit Focus: Recovery/Flexibility

- ☢ Double rope and holding it taunt, stretch from side to side.
- ☢ Double rope twice and "thread the needle" by holding rope out in front as you step one foot through, then the other. Then step feet back out.
- ☢ Back-lying position, put doubled rope around 1 foot, raise leg in air, and gently pull leg towards you for 20 seconds. Repeat with other leg.

Fit Tip

You need to stretch daily. Hold stretches gently for at least 20 seconds.

Fit Session #13

Fit Activity #1   Fit Focus: Agility/Cardiovascular

Agility Course Activities

Use markers such as cones that are easily visible to set up a variety of agility courses.

- ⚽ **Figure-Eight:** Place 2 cone markers about 15 yards/meters apart. Run in a figure-eight pattern around the cones. How many times can your child complete pattern in 30 seconds?

- ⚽ **Triangle Run:** Set cone markers up in a triangular pattern. Number the cones 1, 2, and 3. Have your child start at #1 cone, run around #2, back around #1, then run around #3, back around #1. Repeat this pattern as many times as possible in 30 seconds.

- ⚽ **Garbage Collection Time:** Using hoops or small ropes and beanbags, set up a row of "5 garbage bins" (a beanbag in a hoop), spaced 3 yards/meters apart, in front of a starting line. Have your child run to first bin, pick up beanbag, run back to starting line to place beanbag behind line. Then run to other bins in turn, until all the "garbage" has been collected. Time how long this takes. Repeat activity by putting the garbage out again.

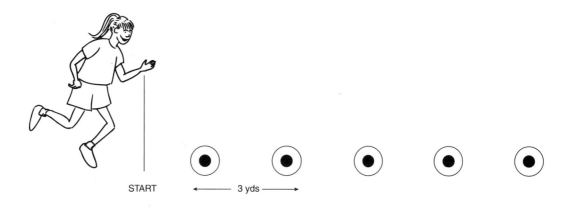

START   ← 3 yds →

Fit Activity #2   Fit Focus: Strength

Tummy Muscle Activities

The following 2 activities strengthen tummy muscles.

- ⚽ **Rope Climbers:** In sitting position, knees raised with weight on heels, lean back and pretend to climb a rope, hand over hand.

- ⚽ **Heel Tappers:** Take weight on your hands and lean back, extend feet out to tap heels in front; then bring legs in to tap heels in close to you.

Leg Muscle Activity

This activity strengthens leg muscles.

- ⚽ **Wall Sit:** Have your child lean with back flat against the wall, then slowly slide down wall until knees are bent at right angles and hold position. Have a conversation with your child as he/she holds this position for 20 seconds. Be sure to give encouragement.

Fit Activity #3   Fit Focus: Flexibility

⚽ **Cross-Leg Stretch:** Sitting against wall, raise one bent leg upwards and gently press towards you for 10 seconds. Change legs and repeat.

⚽ **Calf Stretch:** Have your child stand facing a wall. Lean forward to take weight on hands. Step one leg forward, bending at knee. Keeping back leg straight, press the heel of back foot to floor. Hold for 10 seconds. Repeat with other leg.

Fit Tip

Tummy muscles need to be exercised daily, too. Remember—don't hold your breath when doing a "tummy builder"; breathe regularly.

Fit Session #14

Fit Activity #1   Fit Focus: Cardiovascular

The Family Outing

Just going for a 20–30 minute walk, cycle, swim, skate, and so on with the family is a valuable, socially rewarding activity because it provides the opportunity for the entire family to share the same exercise goal, while reacting socially. Also, this situation will strongly reinforce the concept of fitness for life by showing the child that fitness is a family affair that can be shared and enjoyed by all!

- ⚽ **Walking** with your child and dog around the neighborhood block, park, or beach is a great activity. Do this together at least once a week.

  Set a reasonable distance and gradually increase the distance (time), but remember that children have little legs so there is a limit to the speed you can walk. Better still, "walk and talk" about a favorite subject. Remember to bring a water bottle along with you.

- ⚽ **Hiking or Bush Walking** together in the park or national forest is good exercise and fun! Make it a half or full day's event and end it with a picnic!

- ⚽ **Treadmill Walking or Stepper Walking,** if the weather is not the best for going out-of-doors, is an excellent way to exercise indoors. Use music to move to and try to have your child continue for 15 minutes. Gradually increase time!

Fit Activity #2   Fit Focus: Strength

- ⚽ **Tree Push-Ups:** After completing your walk, find a tree (or similar place), lean forward with hands flat against tree, and bend and strengthen arms to push away from tree. Repeat several times.

- ⚽ **Mountain Sprinters:** Take weight on hands and feet in a front support position (a push-up position), with one leg forward, the other leg back. Exchange leg positions 10 times.

- ⚽ **Stump Step-Ups:** Find a stump or similar place where you can step up and step down from the stump. How many step-ups can you do in 30 seconds?

Fit Activity #3   Fit Focus: Recovery/Flexibility

- ⚽ **Faces:** How many different ways can you make "faces"? Now give me a big smile to relax the muscles in your face. Try these sounds: "Cooo . . . weeee!", "Aaahh!", "Oohh!", "Eeehh!"

- ⚽ **Shoulder Stretch:** Stand tall and reach one hand behind your head and the other hand behind your back. Can you grab the fingers of your hands and hold in this position for at least 10 seconds? Reverse hands and do stretch again.

- ⚽ **Sprinter Stretch:** Begin on all fours. Move 1 leg forward until the knee of the front leg is directly over the ankle, and the other leg is extended back. Hold stretch for 10 seconds. Then gently pulse knee of back leg towards floor. Repeat with other leg.

Fit Tip

Before exercising let your child feel your heart beat and then feel her own. After walking for 20 minutes, let your child again feel your heart beat and tell her why it is faster; then let her feel her own. The muscles are working harder and are hungry for more food and air. This is carried in the blood which the heart pumps around your body. Because your muscles need this nourishment quickly, the heart has to pump quicker.

Fit Session #15

Fit Activity #1   Fit Focus: Cardiovascular

Music Activities

Moving to music (rhythm) can be a life-long, very enjoyable activity. Let your child select a favorite song to play on your tape/CD player.

Have your child move to the music as you give the following signals:

- Clap hands while marching on the spot.
- Jog in place, snapping fingers.
- Bounce on the spot; different ways.
- Skip around the room.
- Hold hands and circle.
- Link elbows and turn one way; other way.
- Slide-step holding hands and "sashay" one direction; return.
- "Jive," turning under each other's arms.
- "Dance" your way to the music.

Fit Activity #2   Fit Focus: Strength

- ⚽ **Hitchhike Walk:** Let your child stand on your feet as you walk around the room. Your child gives you instructions on how to move: 5 steps forward, 8 steps backward, 3 steps to the right, and so on.

    Walk your child to his/her bedroom and say goodnight!

- ⚽ **Inverted Hitchhiker:** Same as "Hitchhike Walk" except that child is upside down, facing you, while you support his/her legs.

- ⚽ Create a Hitchhiker Dance in this position.

Fit Activity #3   Fit Focus: Flexibility

Finger Stretches

For the below exercises, remember to push from the back of the shoulders at same time as fingers are stretching.

- ⚽ Slowly open and close your fingers.

- ⚽ **Spider Push-ups:** press palm of hands together and push fingers away.

- ⚽ Change hand positions: right hand on top; left hand on top; fingers away; fingers up; fingers towards.

- ⚽ Interlock fingers and push away: palms away; palms up.

Fit Session #16

- ⚽ **Tunnel Roll:** Mark 2 lines 10 yards/meters apart. Start at the 1st line. The 1st person rolls the ball backwards between the legs to the 2nd person. The 1st person then runs behind the 2nd person. This repeats until the 2nd line is reached.

  For a challenge see how quickly this can be done or how many times ball gets to 1st person in a given time limit.

- ⚽ **Agility Run & Roll:** Mark off a square that is 5 yards/meters by 5 yards/meters. You stand with a ball in one corner of square; your child stands with a ball in the diagonally opposite corner. On the signal "Roll," each one rolls the ball down the line to the adjacent corner, and then runs to receive the other person's ball and roll it back. Continue in this way.

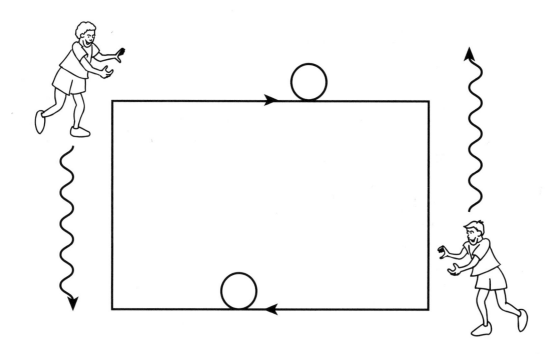

Fit Activity #2   Fit Focus: Strength

⚽ **Hop-A-Long:** Stand side-by-side, holding on at the waist, and hop on outside feet from one line to another line, spaced 5 yards/meters apart.

⚽ **Wheelbarrow:** Stand behind your child, who is on all fours in front of you. Grasp him/her by the upper leg so that child takes weight on hands. Have child walk hands across the floor.

Make sure child does not arch his/her back!

⚽ **Stubborn Mule:** Take up same position as for Wheelbarrow. Ask your child to walk ahead, but offer resistance by not moving with him/her.

Fit Activity #3   Fit Focus: Flexibility

⚽ **Mirrors:** (Use relaxing background music.) Face your child and slowly move stretching limbs in different directions. Your child copies your movements. Switch roles and continue.

⚽ **Huggers:** Hold your child in your arms as you squeeze gently around each other's middle backs.

Now stretch out flat on your back along floor, then sit up to hug knees to chest. Hold in this position for 10 seconds. Slowly breathe in as you stretch flat again; slowly breathe out as you come up to hug knees.

Fit Tip

P.R.I.D.E.   P—Be Positive; R—Be Respectful; I—Intelligent decisions (make good choices); D—Dream; E—Be enthusiastic!

Fit Session #17

Fit Activity #1   Fit Focus: Cardiovascular/Agility

- ⚽ Create an **action poem** and do the actions together:

  Example: Pretend we are going swimming: swimming strokes—front crawl, back crawl; breast-stroking; treading water; butterflying; dog paddling.

- ⚽ **Pantomime** movements such as climbing a ladder; roller-blading or ice-skating (figure-skating); hiking up a mountain; trekking through a tropical jungle; landing on the moon and taking a moon walk; cheer-leading; conducting an orchestra.

- ⚽ Play commercial **dances for children** and together perform the dancing actions such as "Looby Loo," "Little Bird Dance."

- ⚽ Act out movements for **Fairy Tale Classics** such as "Jack and the Beanstalk," "The Three Little Pigs," "Little Red Riding Hood."

Fit Activity #2   Fit Focus: Strength

Create an "Animal Walk Dance" using animal walks such as:

- ⚽ **Puppy Dog:** Walk on all fours.
- ⚽ **Camel Walk:** On your hands and feet, move your right hand and foot, and then your left hand and foot.

- ☺ **Kangaroo Jump:** jump with feet together.
- ☺ **Bunny Walk:** in a squatting position, let hands move forward and then follow with your feet.
- ☺ **Snail Walk:** in a sitting position, slide bottom along floor using legs and hands for support.

Fit Activity #3   Fit Focus: Flexibility

- ☺ **Shakers:** Start with shaking 1 body part; then shake 2 parts; then 3 parts; then 4 parts; 5 parts; 6 parts; all over.
- ☺ **Rockers:** From sitting position, feet together and cross legged, rock forwards and backwards; from side to side; rock up to standing position and stretch high.
- ☺ **Rollers:** Stretch out on your front, and keeping this long pencil shape, roll in one direction; other direction.

Fit Tip

Children love to be creative. Encourage and provide opportunity for their imaginations to be expressed through movement.

Fit Session #18

Fit Activity #1   Fit Focus: Cardiovascular/Agility

Rebounder Activities

A rebounder is a mini-trampoline that can be purchased from a variety of retail stores. Rebound activities are ideal for those days when the weather is not suitable to be outside, and also provide variety in an exercise program. Ensure that the rebounder is located in a safe area, away from any obstacles. Teach your child to enjoy and at the same time, respect the equipment in a safe way! Using music while child is moving on rebounder will enhance rhythm.

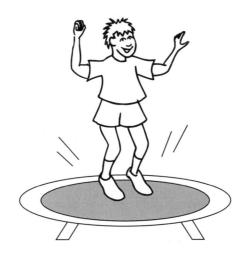

Movements that the parents can call:

- ⚽ Side strides (feet together, feet apart)
- ⚽ Front strides (alternating front and back foot)
- ⚽ Jogging in circle to right; to left
- ⚽ Jumping, keeping knees high
- ⚽ Ski jumping from side to side, feet together
- ⚽ Jumping while crossing one foot in front of other; then behind the other
- ⚽ Jumping to slap heels behind; heels in front
- ⚽ Your turn to create a "rebound" movement!

Fit Activity #2   Fit Focus: Strength/Flexibility

- ⚽ **Roll the Ball:** Have your child sit on the floor in a tightly tucked position like a ball. You sit opposite placing your toes underneath the toes of the "ball" (your child). Try to roll the "ball" by placing pressure under the toes to which the child must resist. Every 20 seconds, you become the "ball" and reverse roles.

- ⚽ **Arm Wrestling:** Lie on fronts facing each other and position right arms at right angles, supporting on the upper arm. Use your other arm to support you as well. Interlock fingers and try to push the other person's hand to the floor.

  (For the wrestling activities the parent should slowly increase the level of resistance and let the child have a "win" now and then.)

⚽ **Leg Wrestling:** Both lie on your backs in opposite directions, hip to hip and interlock legs at the ankle. On signal "Go!", try to push each other's leg to the ground.

Fit Tip

Pain is no gain. Listen to your body. Stretch within your comfortable range of movement.

Fit Session #19

Fit Activity #1   Fit Focus: Cardiovascular/Agility

Dodging Activities

Dodging games have great cardiovascular, agility, and spatial benefits, besides being good fun!

Here are examples of 2 simple Dodging Games that can be played with only 2 or 3 players.

- ⚽ **Wall Dodge:** Use a large soft ball for this activity. Give your child a space which he/she must stay between, then roll the ball towards him/her at a speed he/she can handle. Vary the speed, spin and how you throw it. Children love to think you are trying to trick them, so balk, turn your back on them, and suddenly spin around and throw.

- ⚽ **Dodger in the Middle:** Played with 3 people: 2 rollers or throwers, and 1 "dodger" in the middle.

- ⚽ Get your child to invent a Dodging Game of his/her own and play together, or invent a Dodging Game of your own!

Fit Activity #2   Fit Focus: Strength

- ⚽ **Crab Push-Ups:** Take up a crab-walk position on all fours, face up. Remove 1 arm to tap your bottom, return to place, then repeat with other arm. Continue in this way for as long as you can.

- ⚽ **Finger Push-Ups:** Take up a position on all fours, face down. Lean forward to take weight on hands. Push up onto fingers, then flatten. Continue in this way for as long as you can.

Fit Activity #3   Fit Focus: Flexibility

- ⚽ **Sprinter Stretch:** Sit with 1 leg out straight and the other leg bent in with the foot of the bent leg touching in the inner thigh of the other. Place a small towel or similar length of cloth around the foot of the extended leg and with 2 hands gripping each end of the towel, gently pull back the foot to stretch leg and muscles of the upper back. As your child becomes more flexible, have her hold lower down on towel. Repeat with the other leg extended.

  Hold stretch for at least 10 seconds for each leg. Then repeat 2 more times.

- ⚽ **Knee-To-Nose Touch:** This helps strengthen buttock muscles. Get into an all fours position on hands and knees. Raise 1 leg back and off the floor, keeping it straight and in line with your back. Keep your head straight as well and in line with your back; eyes watching floor. Bend back knee in towards knee and extend. Continue 5–8 times for each knee.

Then stretch back leg over other leg as far as you can and hold this position for at least 10 seconds. Feel the stretch through your seat muscles! Now stretch other leg.

Fit Tip

Always remember to remind your child to bend from the hips and not from the neck.

Fit Session #20

Fit Activity #1   Fit Focus: Cardiovascular/Agility

Tag Belt Chase

You can buy velcro tag belts or simply tuck 2 pieces of cloth into either side of your child's pants or dress.

- ⚽ Start by giving chase. Your child must stop you from stealing the tags by running and dodging away from you. Reverse the roles, but remember that kids love being chased more than chasing!

- ⚽ This activity can be done at different speeds and using different ways of moving: running, brisk walking, skipping, slide-stepping, jumping like a kangaroo.

Fit Activity #2   Fit Focus: Strength

- ⚽ **Seated Wrestle:** Sit side by side with both yours and your child's legs together and out straight. Link closest arms at the elbow and try to roll the other person backwards. The other hand is not allowed to push up from the floor.

- ⚽ **Ball Wrestle:** Hold a soccer ball–size ball in your arms and have your child try to wrestle it away from you.

Fit Activity #3　　Fit Focus: Flexibility

⚽ **Under & Over Stretching:** Stand back to back with your child. Reach under and between your legs and touch hands. Start with your knees quite bent and as flexibility increases complete this activity with the legs straighter. Reach above the head and touch hands. Twist to the left slowly and smoothly, touch hands; repeat to the right.

⚽ Do the above stretch using a ball to pass to each other.

Fit Tip

Make your child as independent as possible. Be there to help your child complete tasks, but encourage independence such as tying shoelaces, dressing himself/herself, and filling up the water bottle.

Fit Session #21

Tag activities/games are always popular with children. Keep the rules simple, but reinforce them. Let your children make up their own rules also.

Fit Activity #1   Fit Focus: Cardiovascular/Balance

- ⚽ **Balance Tag:** Your child runs from you and can be in the "safe" position by performing a balance before being tagged. Have your child practice some of the balances illustrated below, and create a "safe balance" position of his/her own before playing this game.

- ⚽ **Island Tag:** Mark out several 2 yard/meter circles (using rope) or chalk in a 15 meter square play area. These are the "Islands." Your child tries to "swim" from one island to another without getting tagged by the "great white shark" (you, the parent). An island is a safe spot for a 5 second count, then you must leave it.

- ⚽ **Carpet Square Tag:** Carpet squares are inexpensive and can be purchased from Carpet retail stores. Scatter 6 or more squares inside a marked out play area. Play the same way as "Island Tag" or together create your own tag game: Set up different patterns with squares and go "Island hopping" (jumping from 1 square to another!).

Fit Activity #2   Fit Focus: Strength

Stunt Strengtheners

- ⚽ **Bouncing Ball:** Your child is the ball; you are the ball bouncer.
- ⚽ **Scooters:** In sitting position facing your child, hook feet under each other's bottoms. Try to move forwards.
- ⚽ **Rocking Chair:** In same position as for "Scooters," try to rock each other. (You will have to help your child "lift" you!)
- ⚽ **Body Builders:** Facing your child, pretend you are body builders. What different muscle poses can you do?

Fit Activity #3   Fit Focus: Flexibility

- ⚽ **Bear Hug:** Standing tall, lift 1 knee and hug it to your chest. Repeat with the other knee.
- ⚽ **Flamingo Stretch:** You may need to support your child or have them hold onto a table, chair, fence, etc., while he/she balances on 1 foot and grasp the ankle of the other foot. Have child gently pull the foot up to touch the buttocks. Hold for 10 seconds. Repeat with other foot.

Fit Tip

Balances are more stable if the base of support is wider.

Fit Session #22

Balloons are inexpensive, lightweight, manipulative, and great fun. The "slow-motion" quality of the balloons provides success at achieving the task, yet challenges the user.

Fit Activity #1   Fit Focus: Cardiovascular/Agility

Balloon Activities

Clear an area. Mark out a court away from walls and objects that could interfere. Blow up 2 large balloons, 1 for you and 1 for your child.

- Keep your balloon up using different body parts.
- Keep balloon up using only 2 body parts; 3 parts.
- Keep 1 balloon up between the 2 of you using different body parts.
- Use 1 hand to hit, then the other to hit balloon. Keep this order going. Repeat with feet.
- Pretend you are a soccer player and use only your head, knees, or feet.
- Together play "Balloon Volleyball."
- Together play "Balloon Tennis."
- Invent a Balloon Game of your own and play it with a friend!

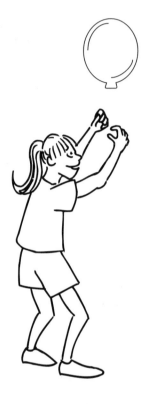

Fit Activity #2   Fit Focus: Strength

⚽ **Balloon Volley:** Using an old sheet, try to shake your balloons off the sheet.

⚽ **Row Your Boat:** Fold the width of the old sheet twice. Sit facing your child; each holds an end. Legs should be bent. While singing "Row, row, row your boat, gently down the stream," pull the sheet to your chest as you rock backwards. (Provide a certain amount of resistance to the child's pull.) Take a "breather" by breathing slowly in and then slowly out, and repeat.

Fit Activity #3   Fit Focus: Flexibility/Cooperation

For these activities you could use a medium-sized beach ball.

- ⚽ **Balloon Pick-Up:** Lie on your tummies, facing each other with balloon placed between you. Using only your heads and working together, slowly lift balloon to the standing position.
- ⚽ **Cooperative Balloon Travel:** Explore different ways of traveling with your balloon using different body parts; for example, hold the balloon between your backs and travel together; or position balloon between your shoulders and travel.
- ⚽ **Balloon Pop:** Using string, tie the balloon to your child's ankle. Then challenge your child to try to "pop" the balloon by stepping on it!

Fit Tip

Remember to "smile" and enjoy your play!

Fit Session #23

Fit Activity #1   Fit Focus: Cardiovascular/Agility

- **Kite Flying:** Take your child to a large open space or playground area or sport oval, void of any electrical wires.

  Of course, you'll need a suitable day for flying your kite. You could even make the kite together, rather than purchase a commercial product.

- **Tire Roll Play:** Pick up a tire from a Spare Parts yard.

  Roll it down a gently sloping area. Give chase.

  Roll the tire back up the hill.

  Roll it so it changes directions.

  Roll it and run around it.

  Can you roll it and safely dive through it?

  Show me other tricks you can do with your tire.

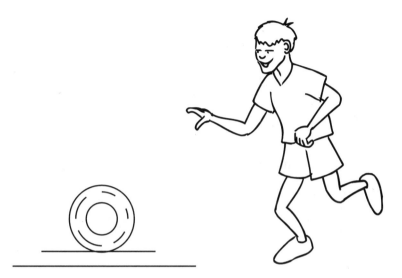

Fit Activity #2   Fit Focus: Strength

- ⚽ Roll the tire back and forth to each other. Stop it first to get control before rolling it back.

- ⚽ Make a bridge over the tire.

- ⚽ Make a bridge on the tire.

- ⚽ Hook your feet under the tire and, keeping your knees bent, do 20 sit-ups.

- ⚽ Jump your feet in and out of the tire.

Fit Activity #3   Fit Focus: Flexibility

⚽ **Shoulder Shrugs:**

Shrug your shoulders up and down.

Roll your shoulders gently backward; then gently forward.

Alternate lifting one shoulder then the other.

Alternate rolling your shoulders backward.

⚽ **Knee Circles:** Keeping your knees close together, circle your knees gently in one direction for 5 circles, then in the other.

⚽ **Ankle Circles:** In sitting position, circle your ankles 5 times in one direction, then circle in the other direction. Point your ankles away from each other, then point your ankles towards you (flex).

Use the cue words: "point"—"flex"—"point"—"flex."

Repeat this pattern 2 more times.

Fit Tip

It is important to keep your ankles strong from an early age. When you are watching TV or during the commercial breaks do some ankle circles!

Fit Session #24

Fit Activity #1 Fit Focus: Cardiovascular/Agility

Bicycling Activities

Insist that your child wear his/her bike helmet at all times while cycling. Attach a water bottle to your bike or carry one in a backpack.

- ⚽ Together with Mom and Dad bicycle in safe areas.
- ⚽ Tricycle or bicycle as Mom (Dad) walks/jogs along.
- ⚽ In an open space such as a parking lot, challenge your child to cycle in a straight line or along marked lines; cycle between markers; cycle around a marked rectangle.
- ⚽ Call out signals: Red Light (stop); Right Turn (signal with right hand and make turn); Left Turn; Yellow Light (Sit on bike and practice looking both ways.)
- ⚽ Bicycle in "slow-motion" from A to B. How slow can you go?
- ⚽ Cycle along designated bicycle paths through the park, along river banks, along beach footpaths.

Fit Activity #2   Fit Focus: Strength/Coordination

When you get to your favorite park or open space:

- Throw a football to each other.
- Throw a Frisbee to each other.
- Kick a soccer ball back and forth.
- Shoot a basketball at a hoop.

Fit Activity #3   Fit Focus: Flexibility

Bicycle Warm-Ups

- **Neck Stretch:** Stretch your neck muscles by gently dropping your head forward and slowly moving it in a half circle to the right and then to the left.
- **Arm Circles:** Circle arms gently backwards.
- **Wing Stretchers:** Gently open and close your arms, keeping your elbows level with your shoulders. Now squeeze your shoulder blades together and hold for 10 seconds. Relax and repeat.
- **Forward Lunge:** (to stretch quadriceps, hip, and thigh muscles). Step forward with right foot, touching left knee to floor. Keep knees bent no more than 90 degrees. Hold for 20 seconds. Repeat with other leg.

Fit Tip

Remember to be a courteous cyclist and obey the traffic rules. Cycle in safe areas!

Fit Session #25

Fit Activity #1　　**Fit Focus: Cardiovascular/Agility/ Balance**

Skating Activities

Where necessary, purchase and insist that your child (and you) wear the proper safety equipment to protect against injury. Participate with your child if you can. Offer encouragement and support to the new learner; otherwise watch and give encouraging smiles!

- ⚽ Take your child ice-skating to an indoor or outdoor rink.
- ⚽ Go roller-blading along the park pathways.
- ⚽ Take your child roller-skating.
- ⚽ There are many games your child can play while doing skating activities, such as:

    "chasey-tag" games

    hockey stick play

    weaving in and out of obstacles

    starting and stopping, turns, and spins

    jumps in the air, jumps off ramps

    create stunts of your own!

Fit Activity #2   Fit Focus: Strength

- ⚽ **Coffee Grinder:** Place one hand on the floor and run your feet around in a circle, in one direction, then the other. Repeat with the other hand.

- ⚽ **Leg Lifters:** In sitting position, lean back and take your weight on your hands. Lift one leg of the floor 5 times; then the other leg. Lift both legs off the floor, spreading legs apart, then together. Make sure you keep hands on floor for support.

Fit Activity #3   Fit Focus: Flexibility

Stick Stretches

Use a hockey stick or a long plastic pole about the same height as your child.

- ⚽ Hold the stick in your hands. Make yourself as long as the stick as you stand on your tip-toes and stretch your arms and hands as high as possible overhead.

- ⚽ Put the stick behind your back, with one hand holding it behind at the lower end, and the other hand holding it at the top end. Gently push forward with the lower hand, to stretch the shoulder of the opposite hand. Hold for 10 seconds, then change hand roles.

- ⚽ Holding stick horizontally above your head, gently stretch to one side and hold for 5 seconds, then to the other side. Push your belly-button out, rather than bending forward so you will get a better stretch.

Fit Tip

First work at achieving good control in the activities you do; then work on speed!

Fit Session #26

Fit Activity #1   Fit Focus: Cardiovascular/Agility/ Strength

---

Wintertime Activities

- ⚽ Make a snowman together, starting with a small snowball and rolling it into a larger and larger snowball. Create a variety of "snow creatures," or "ice sculptures."

- ⚽ Make snow forts and play "Snowball Tag." Remember the most enjoyable play is safe play. Be considerate of others.

- ⚽ Toboggan together on gentle slopes.

- ⚽ Cross-country ski through the park trails.

- ⚽ Downhill ski at local slopes.

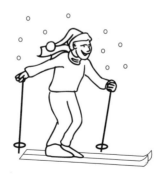

Fit Activity #2   Fit Focus: Flexibility

Ball Massage

This should feel very soothing after an activity session in the snow. Using relaxing background music will help create a pleasant environment.

- ⚽ Have your child lie on his/her stomach and using a tennis ball, roll it over child's legs, back, arms, etc. While massaging with the ball, ask child to close his/her eyes, think happy thoughts, and just relax.

- ⚽ Now ask them to breathe slowly in for 5 seconds; then breathe slowly out for another 5 seconds.

- ⚽ Your turn!

Fit Session #27

Fit Activity #1   Fit Focus: Cardiovascular/Agility

Confined Space Ideas

These activities are great for those rainy days.

- ⚽ **Do This, Do That:** In this activity, the child copies your movement which can be strength, agility, flexibility, cardiovascular, balance, coordination, power, and so on.

  When you say "Do this," the child copies you. When you say "Do that," he/she must not move. Make the changes quickly.

Fit Activity #2   Fit Focus: Alertness

Rocks, Scissors, Paper

This is a reaction game which can be played with 2 or more people.

Hand Motions:

"Rock"—Closed fists, one on top of the other.

"Paper"—One hand flat over closed fist of other.

"Scissors"—Second and 3rd fingers of 1 hand, laid over the closed fist of other hand.

Rules:

To win, rock crushes scissors; paper covers rock; and scissors cuts paper!

Fit Activity #3   Fit Focus: Flexibility / Balance

Limbo

Hold out a long broom handle, or garden stick, or stretch a rope between 2 of you. Challenge child to move under the stick or rope, feet first and face upwards. How low can you go without losing your balance?

Fit Tip

Always bend at your knees to pick up something from a low level, so you don't hurt your back!

Fit Session #28

Fit Activity #1   **Fit Focus: Cardiovascular/Strength/Balance**

Pogo Stick Jumping Activities

You may need to support your child at first until he/she has established a good sense of balance on the pogo stick.

- ⚽ Bounce in a straight line; in a circle; in a square.
- ⚽ Bounce from side to side; forward and back.
- ⚽ Make up a "Pogo stick dance."
- ⚽ Invent other ways of bouncing on your pogo stick.

Fit Activity #2   **Fit Focus: Strength**

More Tummy Muscle Activities

These activities focus on developing strong tummy muscles. They should be done on a comfortable surface such as a mat, carpet, or folded large beach towel. Show your child how to breathe properly: breathing in as she curls up; breathing out as she curls down. Emphasize that she not hold her breath.

- ⚽ **Ankle Tappers:** Begin in back-lying position. Curl forwards to tap your hand to the inside of your opposite ankle. Slowly curl down to lying position. Curl back up and tap with other hand to opposite ankle. Continue in this way.

- ⚽ **Twisting Sit-Ups:** Begin in back-lying position with your knees bent at 90 degrees and fingers at ears. Curl up to touch opposite knee with your elbow; curl down. Then curl back up to touch other knee with opposite elbow. Continue in this way.

Fit Activity #3   Fit Focus: Flexibility

Tension Activities

If possible use soft background music and have your child lie on back and close his/her eyes. Call out different body parts to tighten, then relax:

- ⚽ Tighten toes of left foot (curl toes), then relax.
- ⚽ Tighten toes of right foot—relax.
- ⚽ Tighten tops of legs—relax.
- ⚽ Continue with buttocks; stomach; neck; shoulders; arms; hands and fingers; jaw; eyes.
- ⚽ Tighten up all over!
- ⚽ Then let everything relax like a floppy Raggedy Ann or Andy!

Fit Tip

It is important to balance your play with rest.

Fit Session #29

Fit Activity #1   Fit Focus: Cardiovascular/Agility

- ⚽ **Protected Person:** This is a family activity. Have all but one child join hands and form a circle. The object of the game is for the tagger (child) to quickly run around the outside of the circle and try to tag a nominated person ("Mom"). The circle moves in such a way as to protect the nominated person from the tagger.

- ⚽ **The Family Walk:** This is not your usual way of walking! The family lines up one behind the other to start and then all continue to walk at the same pace, keeping in order, except for the last family member who walks faster or jogs to get to the front of the line. When he/she takes over as the new leader, he calls out "Vitez!" (French for "go quickly"). This is the signal for the last family member to follow pursuit. Decide how many "Vitez" you want to achieve on this walk, and the next walk strive for more!

  You could pick up the tempo and have all family members jog along at a comfortable pace.

  Space family members 1 yard/meter apart and have back runner zigzag run to the front of the file.

Fit Activity #2   Fit Focus: Strength

⚽ **Turn the Turtle:** Have your child lie down on his front and pretend that he is "glued" to the floor. You try to turn him over onto his back. Then exchange roles. Be gentle, but strong as you attempt to turn him over!

⚽ **Knee Wrestle:** Face each other in kneeling position. Interlock hands and try to make the other lose his/her balanced position.

Fit Activity #3   Fit Focus: Flexibility

⚽ **Crab Stretch:** Stand back to back, lean over to grasp each other's hands between your legs. Now try to move in this position forwards, backwards, sideways.

⚽ **Lean Away:** Face your child and, using a wrist grip, have him/her lean away keeping feet touching yours and legs straight. Hold this position as you count to 10 together.

Fit Tip

Make fitness a family affair whenever you can!

Fit Session #30

Fit Activity #1　Fit Focus: Cardiovascular/Agility

Ball Activities

- ⚽ **Family Dodge Ball:** Mark off a large circle using rope or other markers. Have half the family members stand inside the circle, the other half space themselves evenly around the circle. Use a large ball to roll or throw at circle members. If you are successful at hitting a member below the waist, you get to take that person's place in the circle.

- ⚽ **Stinger:** Mark out or designate a large rectangular area. Half the family members are bees with stingers (small softballs). They chase the other family members, throwing the ball to sting them below the knees. If stung, that tagged player becomes a bee and helps to sting other members. All family members must stay inside play area.

  Change game so the bees can take only 3 traveling steps, then they must throw stinger or pass it to another bee to make the tag.

Fit Activity #2　Fit Focus: Strength

- ⚽ **Jump the Ball:** One family member stands in the center and swings a tether ball (ball with rope attached to it) in a large circle along the ground. Other family members must jump over the ball without letting it touch the feet as the ball swings towards her/him. If ball does contact your feet, you must run to touch a designated tree, then you can rejoin the game.

Swing the ball in one direction, then after awhile change directions.

Play so you get 2 "lives" or chances, then the 3rd time you are hit by the swinging ball, you are out.

Gradually raise the ball off the ground, but no higher than knee height.

Fit Activity #3   Fit Focus: Flexibility

- ⚽ **Ball Circles:** Take ball in your hand and trace a large circle. Bend your knees as the ball travels low to ground. Circle 3 times in one direction; then 3 times in the other.

- ⚽ **Ball Leg Roll:** In a sitting position, legs together and stretched out, roll ball from your lap right to your toes, keeping your legs straight. Hold ball on your toes. Stretch ball overhead in lying position and repeat leg roll. Do this 3 times.

Fit Tip

Fit kids have more fun than "couch potatoes!"

Fit Session #31

Fit Activity #1   Fit Focus: Cardiovascular

Pool Activities

- ⚽ **Diving Rings:** These can be purchased from your local pool store or toy store. Scatter rings into the water (at a suitable depth for your child), and have your child dive down to retrieve rings one at a time. Offer praise and encouragement for his/her efforts!

- ⚽ **Floating Rings:** These are large hoop-like rings which will float in the water. Choose the following tasks according to the ability level of your child:

- ⚽ Have your child swim through rings.

- ⚽ Jump into the ring from the edge of the pool.

- ⚽ Swim through 3 rings spaced 1 meter apart from each other.

- ⚽ Hold a ring vertically into water and have your child dive from edge of pool through ring.

- ⚽ Invent your own ring game!

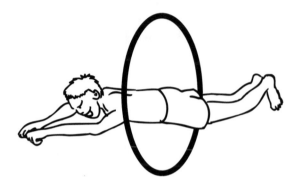

⚽ Play "Pool Tag" in which you are allowed to come out of the pool if being chased, then re-enter somewhere else.

Fit Activity #2   Fit Focus: Strength

⚽ At the beach, walk through knee-deep water.

⚽ Run through knee-deep water.

⚽ Throw a Frisbee or tennis ball to each other in the water.

⚽ Jump over waves.

⚽ Quickly run away so the waves can't "catch" you.

⚽ Dig a large hole or make a sand castle together.

Fit Activity #3   Fit Focus: Flexibility

⚽ Stretch out to the 4 corners of your large beach towel.

⚽ Roll up towel, and stretch it behind your back; then stretch from one side to the other side.

⚽ Make a "sand angel" by lying on your back and opening and closing your arms and legs.

_____

Fit Tip

_____

Remember to wear sunscreen lotion and a hat for protection against the sun's harmful UV rays.

Fit Session #32

Fit Activity #1   Fit Focus: Cardiovascular/Agility

Hoop Activities

Hoops can be purchased at a toy store and provide hours of inexpensive fun.

- ⚽ **Traffic Lights:** Have your child color in 3 large circles each drawn on a piece of thick cardboard: 1 red circle, 1 green circle, and 1 yellow. Mark off a large rectangular area. Have child step inside hoop and hold it at waist height. Hold up sign for child to respond:

  "Green"—run quickly anywhere in the play area.

  "Red"—freeze immediately, then jog in place.

  "Yellow"—use another way of moving such as hopping, skipping, jumping, or walking backwards.

- ⚽ **Dog 'n Bone:** This agility game is best played with 2 children. Mark off 2 lines that are 8 meters (25 ft) apart and place a hoop equal distance between the 2 lines. In the hoop place a beanbag or small ball. Have each child stand just behind his/her line, facing the hoop. On signal "Bone," both children run quickly towards hoop to see which one can get there first to "steal" the bone and take it back to "home" line before being caught by the other "dog."

  Have your children get into different starting positions and watch the fun!

Fit Activity #2   Fit Focus: Strength/Coordination

Hoop Rolling

You may need to initially start rolling the hoop for the child if they are young, but encourage and teach the rolling action to your child as soon as possible.

- Roll your hoop along the ground and run after it to catch it in front of you.
- Roll your hoop and carefully dive through it.
- Roll hoop back and forth to each other.
- Raise and lower hoop overhead and then in front. Continue this pattern 8 times.
- Jump in and out of your hoop with 2 feet; then with 1 foot.
- Skip with your hoop as if it were a jump rope.

Fit Activity #3   Fit Focus: Flexibility

- Show me how you can make your hoop turn around your waist (doing the "hula-hula").
- Hold your hoop horizontally as you stretch from side and hold, then to the other side.
- Hold the hoop in front of you and let your eyes trace its shape in one direction, then in the other.

Fit Tip

Good physical fitness can help you to move safely and to meet unexpected emergencies.

Fit Session #33

Fit Activity #1   Fit Focus: Cardiovascular/Hand-Eye

⚽ **Box the Stocking:** Suspend a ball in a sock or stocking from a clothesline or tree. The ball needs to hang about chest height to your child. Have your child "box" the stocking while moving on the spot for "bouts" of 1 minute. You could even provide a commentary on the action which your child will probably enjoy listening to as he/she boxes away.

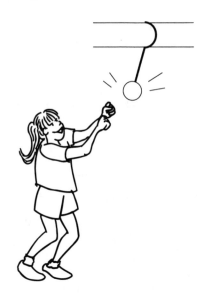

Let him practice his "dancing" footwork as he throws right and left punches into the air.

- ⚽ **Rebound Boxing:** If you have a rebounder available, have child "box" at the stocking while bouncing, "dancing," on the rebounder.

Fit Activity #2   Fit Focus: Strength

- ⚽ **Body Push:** Face each other and touch palm to palm (arms straight). On the count of 3, your child tries to push you backwards as you hold your ground. (Challenge yourself by standing on 1 foot.)

- ⚽ **Foot Push:** Face each other in the sitting position, with the soles of the feet touching. Now try to push against the other's feet.

- ⚽ **Stiff Body Pull:** Face your child who holds his arms rigidly at his sides and makes a fist with his fingers. "Pocketing" his fists in your hands try to lift him upwards. (Remember to bend your knees when lifting!)

Fit Activity #3   Fit Focus: Flexibility

- ⚽ **Music Ball Mirror:** Using music to move to, start in front of your child with each of you holding a small- to medium-sized ball. Begin moving the ball around different parts of the body:

    Back and forth from hand to hand

    Circling around your waist, around your knees, around your ankles

    Moving ball in a figure-eight in and out of your legs

    Circling ball over the head

    Have child simply copy your movements

Fit Tip

Children with movement difficulties often do not learn as well or as quickly as do coordinated children. When explaining an activity to them, keep information simple and easy to follow.

Fit Session #34

Fit Activity #1   Fit Focus: Cardiovascular/Coordination

⚽ **Continuous Rounders:** Set up a "play field" with a rubbish bin/ bucket as the target, and another marker 6 ft (2 meters) to either side. Roll a large ball at the target which the child defends by hitting it with his fist or kicking it. On contact with the ball, the child must then run around the side marker and return to defend the target before the parent retrieves the ball and rolls it at the target. Either as the defender or the thrower, much puffing will be achieved. This would be a great activity for the whole family!

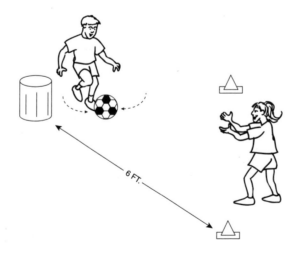

6 FT.

Fit Activity #2   Fit Focus: Strength

- ⚽ **Flying Carpet:** Grab your child with a wrist grip, and gently swing her in a circle around you. Swing in one direction then in the other. You will both probably get dizzy, so break this activity with a "Tightrope Walk."

- ⚽ **Snake Jump:** Using a rope, shake it vigorously along the ground and have your child continually jump to avoid the snake. This needs to be done in short intervals with rest periods in between because fatigue sets in very quickly. Start with 15 seconds of jumping and a 45 second rest. Repeat 4 times. Have your child shake the rope for you so you can try the activity, too!

Fit Activity #3   Fit Focus: Body Coordination

Mirror Activities: Use relaxing background music if possible.

- ⚽ Facing your child and contacting palm to palm, mirror movements such as slow arm circles; raising hands upwards; sideways; downwards.

- ⚽ Other suggestions: body circles; leg lunges. Take turns being the leader.

The main cause of becoming obese results from taking in more calories than are expended. A combination of regular exercise and good eating habits is the most effective way of controlling body fat.

Fit Session #35

Your child will enjoy playing these simple reaction/alertness games.

Fit Activity #1   Fit Focus: Cardiovascular/Agility

⚽ **Hickory, Dickory Dock:** In a large open space, mark out the mouse's home space with a hoop or rope. The child follows the parent around, singing the rhyme, "Hickory, Dickory Dock, the mouse ran up the clock, the clock struck one, the mouse ran down, Hickory, Dickory Dock." Use change of directions, different locomotor movements (walking, running, skipping, slide-stepping, galloping); different speeds. However, when the child hears you whistle or clap, this is the signal for him to quickly scamper home without getting caught. If caught, change roles and continue game in this way.

⚽ **Sock Attack:** Set a certain time limit (2 minutes). Place 2 hoops about 30 ft (10 meters) apart from each other and place 5 beanbags or rolled up socks in each of the hoops. You stand in one hoop; your child stands in the other. On signal "sock attack," pick up 1 sock from your hoop and run to place it in the other person's hoop. Continue in this way until time is up. The object is to have the least number of socks in your hoop.

Fit Activity #2　　　Fit Focus: Reaction

- ⚽ **Quick Hands:** Face your child with your palms up. Child places his hands just over yours, palms down. Child attempts to quickly slap the hands of the parent who moves hands away before the slap. Change roles.

- ⚽ **Quick Tails:** Each tuck a flag in the back of your shorts; about $\frac{2}{3}$ of the tail should be showing. On all fours face each other. Try to grab each other's tails.

Fit Activity #3　　　Fit Focus: Flexibility

- ⚽ **Arm Stretch:** Stand behind child and gently pull arms back and together, squeezing shoulder blades together. Let your child tell you how far to go. Hold for 10 seconds. Repeat.

- ⚽ **Hamstring Stretch:** Stand facing your child who is in a back-lying position with 1 foot raised. Holding this foot, gently push towards your child's head. Keep asking your child when the pressure is just enough, but not painful. (Hamstrings are those muscles located on the back of the upper leg.)

- ⚽ **Side Leg Raises:** Have your child lie on his/her side with the top leg straight and the bottom leg slightly bent. Raise and lower upper leg. Keep knee caps pointing forward. Position just behind your child to ensure that he/she stays off his/her side while doing leg raise. After 10 tries, switch to the other side.

Fit Tip

It is important to dress suitably for exercise. Make sure your child has proper running shoes.

Fit Session #36

Fit Activity #1   Fit Focus: Cardiovascular/Agility

Socktail Play

Place a tennis ball or rolled up socks in an old stocking or long basketball sock to make a "socktail." Knot the stocking at the top of the ball. A commercial product called a "Foxtail" can be purchased from most toy stores.

⚽ Gripping the tail of the stocking, swing it around and around in a large forward arc, and let it go high as possible into the air. Try to catch the socktail as it comes down. How high can your socktail go?

⚽ Swing your socktail and let it go out and up to see how far you can get your socktail to travel. Then run and fetch it.

⚽ Swing your sock and send it back and forth to each other.

⚽ Overhand throw the socktail to each other by grasping the head of the socktail and throwing it.

⚽ Send the socktail back and forth over a low net.

Socktail Volleyball

Play this with the whole family using 2–4 socktails and a volleyball court with a 6 ft (2 meters) net height. Divide the family members into 2 even teams who face each other on opposite sides of the net. Each team has 2 socktails and throw them over the net into the opposition's court. The object of the game is to catch the socktail so it doesn't land on your side of the net; otherwise the other team scores a "socktail point."

Appoint someone on each team to keep score.

Fit Activity #2   Fit Focus: Strength/Body Management

Falling Activities

These activities teach your child how to land safely when falling and prevent injury. Ideally do on a soft surface such as a mat or carpet; otherwise grass will do.

- ⚽ From kneeling position, fall forward. Take your weight on your hands, bending arms to stop you before your stomach touches the mat. Keep your hands flat, fingers slightly inwards, and back straight.
- ⚽ Repeat from kneeling position, fall forward, then roll.
- ⚽ Repeat from a squat position, fall forward; then add roll.
- ⚽ From a standing position, fall forward like a tree. "Timber!"
- ⚽ Repeat "Timber!" and add roll as soon as contact with hands is made.
- ⚽ **Dominoes:** With your family members, kneel beside each other, spaced about 1 meter apart. On the signal "Dominoes," the 1st member falls forward, immediately followed by 2nd; etc.

  Do "Dominoes" from a standing position.

Fit Tip

Children need to learn to make good landings at an early age to absorb force of landing and avoid jarring of body joints!

Fit Session #37

Fit Activity #1   Fit Focus: Cardiovascular/Agility

Frisbees are good fun at any time. Teach your child how to hold and throw a Frisbee, then try this game.

⚽ **Frisbee Golf:** It's recommend that you use the "ring" type Frisbee for young children (easier to throw). Together with your child create and mark out a "golf course" in your neighborhood park or school oval using trees, posts, and other objects as the "holes." Pick your "tee off" spot.

Throw the Frisbee until the target ("hole") is hit. Encourage your child to walk at a good pace or run in between holes. Count the number of throws it takes you to hit the target. You could keep a score card with you and keep track of your overall score.

⚽ **Soccer Golf:** Set up a similar course, but use a soccer ball which is kicked towards target until it is hit.

Fit Activity #2   Fit Focus: Strength/Body Management

More Falling Activities

These activities teach your child how to fall backwards safely to prevent injury. Ideally do on a soft surface such as a mat or carpet; otherwise grass will do.

- ⚽ From a sitting position rock backwards. Let arms take your weight.
- ⚽ From a standing position, squat down and fall backwards, rocking onto your back.
- ⚽ Stand, fall backwards, rock onto your back, rock forwards, and stand again.
- ⚽ Jump up, land bending your knees, rock backwards, rock forwards to stand, and spring upwards again. Repeat.

Fit Activity #3   Fit Focus: Flexibility

Swinging Body Parts

Use music to enhance "swinging parts."

- ⚽ **Head:** nod, shake, gently roll from side to side.
- ⚽ **Shoulders:** shake, shrug, circle.
- ⚽ **Arms:** swing one at a time, backwards and forwards; swing arms together, circling, opening, and closing.
- ⚽ **Legs/Feet:** shaking, bending, lunging; on tip-toes then flat; ankle circling; leg lifts.
- ⚽ **Hands:** fingers opening and closing; making a fist, relaxing; waving; finger snapping; hand clapping; interlocking; pulling against each other.

Fit Tip

"Cooling down" after your heart has been working so hard is important. Remember to breathe normally while stretching; don't hold your breath.

Fit Session #38

Fit Activity #1   Fit Focus: Cardiovascular/Agility

- ⚽ **Give Me Five:** Stand facing your child and hold your hand out in front, palm upwards. Have child run around you a given number of times. Each time they pass you in front, they must give you "Five!" by slapping (gently) the palm of your hand. Have child travel clockwise; then counterclockwise. To give your child a breather, you have your turn!

- ⚽ **Hopscotch:** This is an old favorite and is a great coordination/leg strength activity for children of all ages. Together design your own hopscotch pattern using chalk on tarmac or bright colored floor tape on tiles. Some patterns are illustrated below. With smaller children, the hopscotch spaces will need to be closer together. Use a soft throwing item like a beanbag or a rolled sock. Together make up the rules of your game to allow your child to experience success. Above all, play yourself! Cognitive variations may include using letters, shapes, or colors instead of numbers.

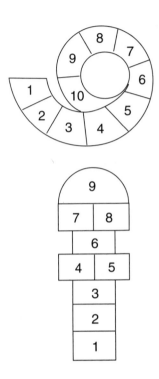

Fit Activity #2   Fit Focus: Strength/Body Management

Sideways Falling Activities

- ⚽ From a kneeling position, fall sideways to rock onto your arm first, then side, and shoulder. Fall sideways in one direction, then in the other.
- ⚽ Fall down a grassed slope rolling sideways.
- ⚽ From a standing position, do a forward shoulder roll: roll onto your lower arm, then upper arm, shoulder, back, and up onto your feet.

Shake Hands Partners

- ⚽ Face each other in a front support position and lift right hands to shake.
- ⚽ Shake left hands.
- ⚽ Challenge: Try to pull each other off balance!

Fit Activity #3   Fit Focus: Flexibility

- ⚽ **Arm/Shoulder Stretch:** Cross-leg sit "tall" on floor. Raise one arm so that hand is touching your upper back. Use other hand to press gently down on the raised arm's elbow. Feel the stretch of your tricep muscles (underneath upper arm) as you hold for 10 seconds. Reverse arms and repeat stretch.

- ⚽ **Knee Rolls:** Sit on the floor with legs bent and arms supporting behind the body. Keep your knees together as you roll them to touch the floor on the right; then touch on the left. Remember to keep both hands on the floor.

Fit Session #39

Fit Activity #1   Fit Focus: All-Around Workout

Obstacle Course Activities

These are readily available in many parks and school grounds, but they can also be easily set up at home. The idea of an obstacle course is to repeat the course a set number of times and within a time limit. The challenge is therefore to beat the number of course completions or to beat the clock.

Here is an example of a home obstacle course:

- ⚽ Climb a fence.
- ⚽ Run to the corner of the yard.
- ⚽ Walk across the bridge without falling in (4' × 2" length wooden beam).
- ⚽ Hand to hand travel between or on the rungs of a ladder.
- ⚽ Hop between the markers.
- ⚽ Rope climb up to a knot. (Rope suspended from a sturdy tree branch.)
- ⚽ Hang from a narrow beam.

On the next page is an obstacle course card you can copy and use to record and note improvements. (Or, design your own with your child.)

Obstacle Course Card

Age:	Weight:	Height:

Date:	Activity:	Target Number:	Time:

Fit Tip

You and your child could create your own obstacle course that could be set up in a rumpus room in your house, using chairs, tables, carpet squares, ropes, hoops, cushions, poles, music, and so on.

Fit Session #40

You can produce simple circuits in the home and together with your child through a number of activities. Music can be used to enhance the circuit activities and for timing. The idea of a circuit is that your child can either complete a certain number of attempts for each activity in a given target time or as fast as possible. Alternatively, your child can work for a set time and complete as many attempts as possible for each activity. The target numbers should be obtained through initially observing how many trials can be completed in a set time, and then trying to better the score for that particular activity.

Fit Activity #1 **Fit Focus: Cardiovascular/Strength/ Agility/Balance**

Indoor Circuit

Following is an example of a 5-station indoor circuit that you could do with your child. You do not need a lot of space; a normal room provides ample space.

- ⚽ **Rebound Jogging:** Jog lightly on rebounder.
- ⚽ **Drop and Pick:** Drop a sock or beanbag behind you. Reach between your legs to pick it up.
- ⚽ **Partner Throw:** Pass a ball back and forth to each other as many times as you can in the time limit.
- ⚽ **Circle Walk:** In a front support position, keeping your feet in the same spot, make a circle by walking around with hands.

⚽ **Under the Bridge:** Have your child in a seated position with legs out in front and bent at the knees. Your child must maneuver a large ball around her body without moving her bottom. Try having your child pass the ball under the legs while holding them off the ground.

Sample Circuit Record Card:

Nikki's Circuit Card		
Age:	Weight:	Height:
7	45 lbs	3'10"

Date:	Activity:	Target Number:	Time:
3/6/96	Rebound Jog		2 mins
	Drop & Pick	5 either side	1 min
	Partner Throw	20	2 mins
	Circle Walk	3	1 min
	Bridge	8	1.5 mins

On the next page is a circuit card you can copy and use to record and note improvements. (Or, design your own with your child.)

Circuit Card			
Age:	Weight:		Height:

Date:	Activity:	Target Number:	Time:

Fit Tip

When doing circuits you cannot expect to improve every time. You should explain to your child that sometimes they may not perform as well as the time before. This can be due to being tired, or not feeling well on one day; but they could do extra good on another day. Over time, improvement will occur.

Fit Session #41

Fit Activity #1   Fit Focus: All-Around Workout

Outdoor Circuit

Below are suggestions for setting up a 5-station outdoor circuit. Have your child move against a set time or repeat an activity a certain number of times. There are several other fitness activities in this book that can be incorporated into similar circuits.

Some fitness activities that can be incorporated into similar circuits are:

Balloon activities (page 67)

Ball activities (page 87)

Pool activities (pages 89)

Hoop rolling (page 93)

Frisbee activities (page 106)

⚽ **Locomotion Rectangle:** Mark out a rectangle 15 yards/meters by 10 yards/meters. Your child moves around the sides of the rectangle using different forms of locomotion. Set up a corner sign to indicate the type of movement to be used.

For example:

- ⚽ Run forwards down (side 1)
- ⚽ Hop along the width (side 2)
- ⚽ Skip down (side 3)
- ⚽ Walk backwards along width (side 4)

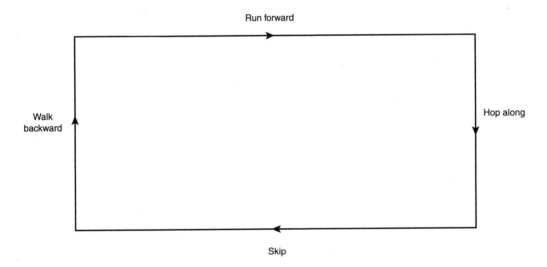

Run forward

Walk
backward

Hop along

Skip

- ⚽ **Ball Swat:** From a squatting position, your child jumps up as high as possible to try to swat a ball in a hanging stocking. Earn a point each time you slap the ball. Remind your child to bend his knees on each landing!

- ⚽ **Skipping:** Jump rope for a set number of times, or skip from a starting line to a turning line and back.

- ⚽ **Beat the Clock:** Mark out the center and 6 o'clock positions around the circle. Your child must run to touch each marker and then back to the center of the circle.

- ⚽ **Beam & Crab Walk:** Have your child walk along a beam (2' × 4" wood) from one end to the other, jump off the end and crab walk back to the start of the beam. (Crab Walk is done by having child lift himself from a seated position and use his hands and feet to move forwards or sideways.)

Fit Tip

Always try to ensure the safety of your child. Teach him to be aware of moving safely and to respect the equipment he is using.

Fit Session #42

Fit Activity #1   Fit Focus: All-Around Workout

Trampoline Activities

If you have a trampoline in your back yard or access to one in another way, the trampoline can be used to strengthen leg muscles as well as improve aerobic capacity.

Emphasize that your child stay in the center on the trampoline; do a safety jump to stop movement; only 1 person on the trampoline at a time; and get off carefully. The trampoline should have safety pads around all the sides. Mark an "X" in the center of the tramp with chalk. Ensure that your child takes little "stretching breaks," as this is quite a strenuous activity.

Have your child do the following tasks:

- ⚽ Do little bounces up and down on the "X" spot, bending at your knees. Look straight ahead, and make circles with your arms as you jump upwards.
- ⚽ Bounce while clapping your hands; snapping your fingers.
- ⚽ Stop by bending at your knees, feet shoulder width apart, and arms held sideways for balance.

- Bounce again, gradually see how high you can bounce.
- Bounce and turn in a circle, one direction; other direction.
- Bounce onto your knees and back up to your feet.
- Bounce onto your seat and back up to your feet.
- Can you bounce from knees, to seat, to feet?
- Bounce with your feet together, feet apart; bounce changing front foot.

Trampoline Challenges

- Do quarter-jump turns (90 degree turns); half-jump turns (180s); three-quarter-jump turns; full turns (360s)
- Have your child bounce on the trampoline while catching a ball and throwing it back to you. Have them try to skip with a short rope.
- Bounce on trampoline while tossing and catching a ball.
- Bounce to touch your toes in front; heels behind you.
- What other stunts can you do?
- Lie down on the trampoline and stretch out wide and hold for 10 seconds; curl up into a ball and stay for 10 second count; grasp your ankles with your feet in the air and hold for 10 seconds.

Fit Tip

In choosing the location for the trampoline, be sure there are no dangerous objects near it.

Fit Session #43

Not all activities need to involve children running, jumping, and so on. As we stated earlier, coordination is often the key that unlocks the door to activity and fitness. This is why you need to mix the fitness sessions mentioned with skill development. The next 5 sessions will give you ideas of activities that will promote coordination which will in turn assist in fitness development in the long term.

Fit Activity #1   Fit Focus: Hand-Eye Coordination

- ⚽ **Rolling Soccer:** Using some kind of marker like cones, cans, or bricks, make goals that are 3 yards/meters apart and position just in front of a wall. Have partners take turns being the roller who stands 4 yards/meters away from the wall and tries to roll a ball between the goals. The other partner is the goalie who uses his feet to protect the goal and stop goals from being scored. Use a ball suitable for the age ability of your child.

- ⚽ **Home Hockey:** Set up a goal as for "Rolling Soccer." Each partner has a hockey stick. One partner is the scorer; the other partner is the goalie. Use a tennis ball or other type of soft ball to score goals.

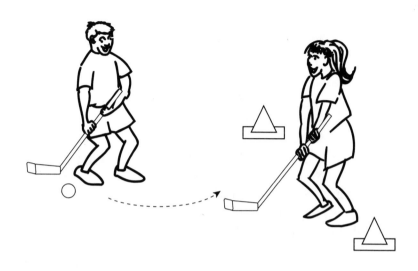

Fit Session #44

Fit Activity #1   Fit Focus: Hand-Eye Coordination

⚽ **Bowling Roll:** Mark a line and place 3 plastic jugs about 5 yards/ meters away. Arrange the jugs in a pyramid fashion. Have your child roll the ball towards the jugs trying to knock them over. Increase rolling distance as "bowling" skill is mastered.

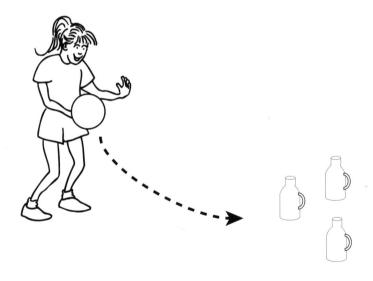

⚽ **Wall Bounce:** Stand facing a wall with your child. Toss a ball at the wall and have your child catch it after one bounce off the ground. Repeat. Offer challenges such as "clap" hands before catching ball; "snap" fingers; "touch" your shoulders before catching; turn around once; and so on.

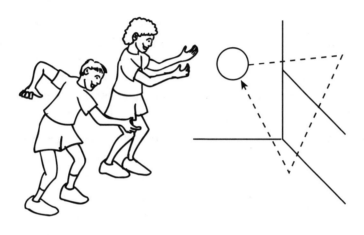

Fit Tip

Remind your child often to keep his/her eyes on the "target." Catch with "soft" hands, keeping fingers relaxed. Let the throwing hand follow through in the line of direction.

Fit Session #45

Fit Activity #1   Fit Focus: Hand-Eye Coordination

⚽ **One Step Back:** Start 3 giant steps away from your child. Throw the ball to your child. Make 3 successful catches, then have child take 1 step away from you. Continue in this way.

⚽ **Obstacle Bouncing:** Using hoops, cones, or chairs, scattered around the play area, have your child follow you as you each bounce your ball between the obstacles. Start with a 2-handed bounce, then progress to a 1-handed bounce. Start slowly with obstacles far apart. Gradually increase the speed. Then decrease the space in between the obstacles.

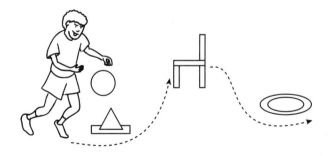

Fit Session #46

Fit Activity #1   Fit Focus: Hand-Eye Coordination

- ⚽ **Ten Pin:** Using 10 plastic milk bottles set up the ten pin bowling formation and play to the same rules as for ten pin bowling. (Bowling sets can also be purchased from toy stores.)

- ⚽ **Horseshoes:** You may have a "Horseshoe Set" which includes 2 pegs and 2 horseshoes. Space the pegs about 3 or 4 yards/meters apart and secure into the ground. Adjust distance to suit the skill level of your child. Each player has a horseshoe. Standing behind one of the pegs, each player in turn tosses a horseshoe towards peg to see who can get it the closest. Play to 10 points.

  Variation: Use a throwing ring and 2 beanbags.

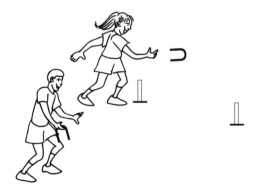

Fit Session #47

Fit Activity #1   Fit Focus: Hand-Eye Coordination

Choose 1 or 2 of the games below and make it your FIT session. Try to include as much running as possible in these games.

- ⚽ **Partner Hit:** With a partner, each holding a racquet, hit a balloon back and forth. How many hits in a row can be made? Hit a ball back and forth to each other, let ball bounce once before hitting it back.

- ⚽ **Box Toss:** Have your child toss a ball or beanbag into a large cardboard box or plastic pail or bin placed near a wall. Gradually increase the distance as throwing skill improves. Use the underhand throw, then the overhand throw. Throw with best hand, then use the other hand.

  Variation: Hit the ball off wall to rebound it into a cardboard box or bin.

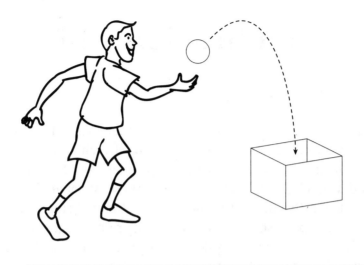

Fit Tip

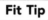

Encourage your child to invent a FIT GAME of his own and play it with him!

Fit Session #48

Although we have included many flexibility exercises in the sessions, you will have noticed that not many are the form of stretching exercises with which your may be familiar. You may wish to do some more formal stretching exercises with your child. We encourage you to do so! What needs to be brought to your attention is that there are some ways of stretching that should be avoided.

Some of the exercises we did as children are no longer recognized as suitable. In fact some are now considered dangerous. The next 3 sessions will provide you with some of the more common stretches.

Stretching Activities

Name of Old Exercise	Why Exclude?	Alternative
1. Side bends standing and seated	Bad for the middle and lower back.	Lie on your back with arms above head. Bend gently to side.
2. Straight leg toe touch—standing and seated	Tears the muscles at the back of the upper leg and	Sit on floor with legs straight and arms supporting from behind.

Name of Old Exercise	Why Exclude?	Alternative
	lower back muscles.	Place both hands on outstretched leg and slowly and gently slide your hands up your leg until you feel a slight stretch. Hold for 5 seconds. Repeat 5 times.
3. Hurdle stretch	Strains the ligaments of the knee that is bent.	Lie on your back with legs straight. Pull knees slowly and gently up to the chest with hands. Hold for 5 seconds.

Fit Session #49

Stretching Activities

Name of Old Exercise	Why Exclude?	Alternative
1. Alternate toe touch	Lower back damage, especially if not fit.	From seated position with legs bent, keeping back straight, alternately touch hand to toes of opposite leg.
2. Straight leg sit-ups	Bad for lower back. Does not strengthen stomach muscles sufficiently.	Bent leg sit-ups with arms folded across chest. Keep back straight. Need not come up all the way.
3. Leg raises holding legs off the ground	Can cause too much pressure on the discs. Is not good for the stomach.	Lie on back with knees bent and arms to the side. Slowly and gently bring both knees up until kneecaps point straight to the sky.

Fit Session #50

Stretching Activities

Name of Old Exercise	Why Exclude?	Alternative
1. Push-ups that sag	Can cause too much pressure on discs in back. Ineffective for improving upper body strength.	Start with a half push-up from the kneeling position, with knees straight under seat. As strength improves move knees further back until a full push-up position is achieved. Remember, no sag.
2. Banana bends lying on stomach holding ankles and pulling them up towards head	Hyperextension of the back.	Lie on stomach with hands under chin and legs stretched and together. Slowly and gently raise one leg at a time to a point where a slight stretch is felt. Hold for 5 seconds.

continues

Name of Old Exercise	Why Exclude?	Alternative
3. Over-the-head toes to touch ground	Can cause damage to the neck.	In standing position, hold your hand against side of head. Push against hand slowly; hand giving resistance. Repeat with hand on forehead.
4. Star jumps	Stress on all joints.	Walk!

136 Notes

138 Notes

140   Notes

142   Notes

144 Notes